ENDOMETRIOS

ENDOMETRIOSIS AND FIBROIDS

The complete guide to the causes, the symptoms and the treatments

Dr Sarah Brewer

with the National Endometriosis Society

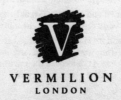

VERMILION

LONDON

DEDICATION
This booklet is dedicated to every woman, everywhere, who has ever suffered from endometriosis.

1 3 5 7 9 10 8 6 4 2

Text copyright © Dr Gail Darlington and Linda Gamlin 1996

The right of Dr Sarah Brewer to be indentified as the author of this book has been asserted by them in accordance with the Copyright, Designs and Patents Act, 1988.

First published in the United Kingdom in 1995
This edition published in 1998 by
Vermilion, an imprint of Ebury Press

Random House
20 Vauxhall Bridge Road
London SW1V 2SA

Random House Australia (Pty) Limited
20 Alfred Street, Milsons Point, Sydney,
New South Wales 2061, Australia

Random House New Zealand Limited
18 Poland Road, Glenfield,
Auckland 10, New Zealand

Random House South Africa (Pty) Limited
Endulini, 5A Jubilee Road,
Parktown 2193, South Africa

Random House UK Limited Reg. No 954009

A CIP catalogue record for this book is available from the British Library

ISBN: 0 09 181649 1

Typeset by Deltatype Limited, Ellesmere Port, Cheshire

Printed and bound in Great Britain by
Cox & Wyman Ltd, Reading

Papers used by Random House UK Limited are natural, recyclable products made from wood grown in sustainable forests. The manufacturing processes conform to the environment regulations of the country of origin.

CONTENTS

ACKNOWLEDGEMENTS AND THANKS

I would like to thank the various experts who kindly gave so much of their time to check the manuscript and add helpful comments. In particular, I would like to thank Diane Carlton and Dr B.I. Pirzada of the National Endometriosis Society, and Dr Andrew Prentice of The Rosie Maternity Hospital, Cambridge.

As always, grateful thanks to my agent, Serafina Clarke, and to the best authors companion and aide in the world, Richard Marchant.

FOREWORD

Endo WHAT? is the typical response when the word endometriosis is first mentioned. The disease is also embarrassing to explain, painful to live with and problematical to treat. It can also have a profound effect on a woman's quality of life, and can disrupt her career. Feelings of isolation and despair are often expressed by the sufferers due to the effects of their pain and/or treatments, and in some cases the trauma of infertility.

Often described as the enigmatic disease, endometriosis can mimic other medical problems by producing symptoms similar to irritable bowel syndrome, pelvic inflammatory disease and cystitis. Consequently, it may be initially misdiagnosed. In a survey conducted by the Society amongst 2,102 of its members, the average delay in diagnosis was shown to be 6–8 years. Distressingly, nearly a quarter of the women surveyed had suffered for ten years or more before diagnosis, and a few women – some 4% – had experienced a delay of 20 years.

This book will enable sufferers and others interested in the disease to understand more about endometriosis, fibroids and their effect on a woman's well-being. More importantly, it will help women make an informed choice regarding the treatment available.

Dr Sarah Brewer has worked closely with the National Endometriosis Society in the writing of this book. The Society is certain that it will go a long way towards promoting a better understanding of endometriosis and fibroids, and would like to thank Dr Brewer for writing a book which is so distinguished and informative.

Diane Carlton
Chair to the Board of Trustees,
and to the Medical Panel
The National Endometriosis Society

INTRODUCTION

Endometriosis is something of a medical conundrum. It is the only known condition in which normal, non-cancerous calls spread from one part of the body to another, take root and continue to grow.

Usually, the spreading of tissues from one part of the body to another is linked with a major cell abnormality and results in a serious illness such as cancer. In endometriosis, however, the displaced cells involved are only slightly different from normal endometrial cells and are certainly not cancerous.

Endometriosis occurs mainly in women of reproductive age. Because the cells involved are physiologically active and continue to respond to a woman's menstrual cycle, they cause problems at certain times of the month. A few women have problems all the time.

Despite the fact that endometriosis is surprisingly common, and despite intensive scientific and clinical research into the nature of the disease, its cause remains a mystery. Recent advances in drug treatment, however, are a major step forward in relieving the symptoms of many sufferers.

WHAT IS ENDOMETRIOSIS?

Like many medical words, the term *endometriosis* is derived from the ancient Greek:

- *end* means 'inside',
- *metra* means 'womb',
- *osis* means 'disease, problem or abnormality'.

The endometrium is therefore the inside lining of the womb, while endometriosis means an abnormality or problem connected with it. This problem can be summed up as the presence of endometrial (womb lining) cells in an unusual site outside the womb cavity. This displaced tissue is known as ectopic (outside its normal site) endometrium.

The most common place where ectopic endometrial cells are found is in the abdominal cavity, either on the membrane lining the cavity (peritoneum) or on the outer surface of the pelvic organs or intestines. Ectopic endometrial cells can also travel farther afield, and have been found in the lungs, nose, ears and even behind the eyes.

Endometrial tissues are programmed to respond to a woman's hormonal cycle. Displaced endometrial cells are no exception, and continue to show some response to a woman's hormones. Some of the ectopic cells swell up at the same time as those found in the normal endometrium, and some will bleed into surrounding tissues when menstruation occurs each month. This ectopic bleeding into previously healthy tissues triggers an enzymatic response and results in a build-up of inflammation and scarring. This process produces fluid-filled hollow cysts (vesicles) and solid nodules of varying size. Those that form on the ovaries are often referred to as chocolate cysts because of their colour. This colour is due to the action of enzymes acting on red blood and changing it into a thick, dark-brown sludge.

All this inflammation can cause structures such as the bowel and bladder to become matted together in a web of scar tissue, and in many cases intense, long-term (chronic) pain may develop. This often makes intercourse painful or downright impossible. Scarring can also interrupt the normal function of the bowel, bladder, ovaries and Fallopian tubes and can affect fertility.

Endometrial cells can also be found trapped inside the muscular walls of the womb itself. This is called adenomyosis (see page 34). When these cells respond to the female hormonal cycle, bleeding between muscle fibres can cause distension and severe pain and may also trigger overgrowth of surrounding muscle.

· *How common is it?* ·

Endometriosis is the second most common gynaecological condition after fibroids. It is seen most frequently in women between the ages of 25 and 40 but can affect any woman from the onset of her periods (menarche) to the menopause – and sometimes beyond.

It is currently estimated that around 10 per cent of women are affected. This can be further broken down into specific groups:

● Between 2 and 5 per cent of healthy women of childbearing age, who have already had a pregnancy (i.e. proven fertility) have some degree of endometriosis, although many women do not notice any symptoms and it may be diagnosed only if surgery is required for another condition.

● Of those women who do have pelvic pain and who undergo a diagnostic laparoscopy (keyhole telescopic investigation of the female reproductive organs), endometriosis is confirmed in 10–15 per cent.

● In women undergoing investigation for subfertility, endometriosis is diagnosed in 30–40 per cent of cases. It is more common in these women because the inflammation and scarring associated with endometriosis can cause infertility.

These figures are probably an underestimate. They are based on visual evidence of the classic, pigmented deposits characteristic of endo-metriosis. New research suggests that many more women with atypical, non-pigmented lesions have previously escaped diagnosis because their lesions look so different (see page 29). Even more women who are experiencing infertility may have microscopic deposits of endometriosis that do not show up on visual inspection and are found only on microscopy of healthy-looking tissues (see page 30).

If these atypical cases are taken into account, and if a chemical or immunological diagnostic test for endometriosis is developed, it is likely that at least 20 per cent of women – twice the current estimate – would be found to have endometriosis.

Not surprisingly, endometriosis has been diagnosed more frequently since the introduction of laparoscopy. Before then, cases were diagnosed through a combination of clinical alertness to symptoms and signs and, occasionally, an open operation (laparotomy). Laparoscopy provides a less invasive, relatively safe method of visually inspecting the pelvic organs. The diagnosis of endometriosis at laparoscopy increased from 42 per cent in 1982 to 72 per cent in 1988. The greatest change was in the detection of atypical, subtle lesions, which increased from 15 per cent in 1986 to 65 per cent in 1988.

2

THE FEMALE
REPRODUCTIVE TRACT

The way the reproductive tract develops in a female embryo is fascinating. It's worth reading about these events so that you can understand:

- why some of the theories on the cause of endometriosis have been suggested
- why some theories on the origin of endometriosis are unlikely
- why endometriosis can occur in men under certain rare conditions.

· Determining the baby's sex ·

The sex of an embryo is determined at the time of fertilisation. Each egg contains a single female sex chromosome (X). Each sperm contains either a female sex chromosome (X) or a male sex chromosome (Y). If a female sperm (X) fertilises the egg (X), a female embryo (XX) results. If a male sperm (Y) fertilises the egg, a male embryo with XY sex chromosomes results.

In a female embryo, the female reproductive cells (eggs, or ova) are made in a process called oogenesis.

· The Ovaries ·

The sex glands develop from an area called the genital ridge on each side of the embryo. Each gland develops an outer part, called the cortex, and an inner part called the medulla. Until the sixth week of development, the sex glands in both sexes are identical.

Then, beginning in the seventh week, sexual differentiation begins to take place.

- In the male, the medulla develops into the testis during the seventh and eighth weeks and the cortex regresses. The testis starts secreting the male hormone, testosterone, until after birth, when secretion stops, to be resumed at puberty.
- In females, the cortex develops into an ovary and the medulla regresses. The ovary does not secrete female hormones until puberty.

· *Egg production* ·

Each baby girl is born with her full complement of eggs. These lie dormant until activated in a menstrual cycle at puberty and continue to be released until the menopause. After the menopause, no further egg cells will be activated and released. This is very different from the male, who does not produce any sex cells until puberty, and then continues making new sperm throughout his adult life.

The ovaries start to develop early in the first few weeks of life. Germ cells (oogonia) mature and develop so that by the third month after conception, the developing baby girl has 7–8 million immature eggs divided between her two ovaries. Each immature egg is protected by a tiny nest of cells called a primary follicle. The cells surrounding each follicle are full of tiny granules, rich in cholesterol, which will produce the female hormones, oestrogen and progesterone, at puberty.

During the fifth and sixth months of the fetus's development, most of these egg follicles start to break up and are reabsorbed; why this happens is unknown.

- A five-month-old female fetus contains about 7 million immature eggs.
- By the time of birth, around 2 million follicles are present, but half of these are regressing.
- At puberty, only 40,000–400,000 primary follicles remain.

· *The Mullerian ducts* ·

In the seventh week of development, the embryo has both male and female primitive genital ducts, the Mullerian and the Wolffian systems.

- In the female, the Mullerian ducts develop into the uterine (Fallopian) tubes and the uterus, while the Wolffian ducts regress.
- In the male, the Wolffian ducts develop into the sperm-carrying tubes (epididymis and vas deferens) while the Mullerian ducts regress.

The Mullerian ducts appear as two vertical tubes on the back wall of the abdominal cavity, one on each side, during the sixth week of an embryo's development.

In a female embryo, these tubes grow downwards and in towards the middle, where their bottom ends fuse. This forms a Y-shaped tube, with two arms that will form the Fallopian tubes, and a fat tail that will develop into the uterus.

In a male embryo, the Mullerian ducts also start to grow, but they wither away during the third month of development once the male testes produce testosterone and a protein known as Mullerian-inhibiting substance (MIS). The ducts leave behind two remnants:

● The top end of each arm of the Y-shaped duct leaves a little structure above the testicle called the appendix of the testicle.

● The bottom end of the duct forms a tiny anatomical pit in the tube passing from the male bladder, through the penis to the outside world (urethra). This pit, which represents the closed-off bottom end of the Mullerian duct, is found in the part of the urethra passing through the prostate gland and is known as the prostatic utricle. In rare cases, men receiving hormone treatment for advanced prostate cancer have been found to have endometriotic tissue, and this is thought to come from the vestiges of the Mullerian duct(s).

· *The Fallopian tubes* ·

Each Fallopian tube develops from one of the arms of the Y-shaped Mullerian duct once it has fused. During the fourth and fifth month of development, the tube grows rapidly and becomes coiled. A thick, muscular wall and the mucous membrane lining of that wall develop.

The upper end of each Fallopian tube swells and develops a number of finger-like projections called fimbriae. These are important in catching an egg once it is released from an ovary.

The lining of the adult Fallopian tube contains cells with small, hair-like projections called cilia. These wave around to set up eddy currents in the fluid within the tube. The cilia help to carry a newly ovulated egg downwards to the womb. Eddy currents in the fluid help to transport sperm upwards.

· *The Uterus* ·

The pear-shaped uterus forms from the lower, fused ends of the two Mullerian ducts. The fusion between the two ducts is at first incomplete, and a thin membrane (septum) separates the developing womb into two cavities. The septum then usually disappears, leaving a single cavity. The angle where the two arms of the Mullerian ducts join grows to form a convex dome which becomes the upper part (fundus) of the womb.

The wall of the uterus thickens up and becomes muscular, while the lowest end develops into the cervix.

The cavity of the womb is lined with immature endometrial tissue. As the Fallopian tubes and womb have both developed from the Mullerian tubes, the cells lining the womb and tubes are continuous and were once identical. For some reason, the cells lining the Fallopian tubes go on to mature into ciliated mucous cells, while those lining the uterus go on to develop into endometrial tissues.

· *The Vagina* ·

The vagina forms from a different embryonic tissue from that which forms the uterus. Once the solid end of the fused Mullerian ducts (immature cervix) develops, it stimulates formation of a flat, circular collection of cells called the vaginal plate. These rapidly thicken and grow downwards to form a solid cylinder. This starts to hollow out during the eleventh week of development. By the fifth month, the vagina is fully formed, and the lower end of the hollow tube remains as a thin, incomplete membrane called the hymen.

Possibly because the vagina develops from a different type of embryonic tissue from that of the womb and cervix, it largely seems to escape involvement with endometriosis in later life.

· *The Vulva* ·

The external genitals start to develop during the seventh week of development from a structure called the genital fold. At the top end, a small lump enlarges to form the clitoris, while two folds appear around the lower end of the developing vagina to form the vaginal lips (inner, labia minora, and outer, labia majora).

· *The Peritoneal membrane* ·

The peritoneal membrane, which lines the abdominal cavity, has been intensively investigated, as its cells may possibly undergo changes and act as a source of ectopic endometrial cells.

The embryonic tissue that develops into the peritoneal membrane (the coelomic or peritoneal mesenchyme) starts development as a small pouch on the right side of where the oesophagus (gullet) eventually lies. This pouch grows upwards, into the future chest cavity, and downwards into the future peritoneal cavity. These two areas are then separated by the developing diaphragm.

If endometriosis were caused by cells present in the peritoneal membrane, they might be expected to occur as frequently in the chest cavity as well, yet they do not.

3

THE MENSTRUAL CYCLE

A woman's menstrual cycle is controlled by a series of hormones known as the hypothalamo-pituitary-gonadal axis. This is rather a mouthful, but basically means that the hormones involved come from three sites, the pituitary gland, a part of the brain just above it (hypothalamus) and the ovaries (female gonads).

The pituitary gland releases two hormones concerned with female reproduction. These are:

- follicle-stimulating hormone (FSH)
- leutinising hormone (LH).

These two hormones are together known as gonadotrophins as they work on the gonads (the testicles in males and the ovaries in females). They tend to be released in short pulses throughout the day and night, rather than at a steady level. Release of these two gonadotrophins is controlled by a hormone secreted in the hypothalamus which is also released in intermittent short pulses. This control hormone is called Gonadotrophin Releasing Hormone – or GnRH for short.

Puberty – the start of the menstrual cycle

At puberty, the ovaries are switched on by increasing amounts of FSH and LH released from the pituitary gland under the control of GnRH.

The awakened ovaries start to make the female hormones, oestrogen and progesterone, and these, together with other hormones such as growth hormone, thyroid hormone and adrenal gland hormones, trigger the physical changes of puberty.

The first period (menarche) usually occurs between the ages of 10 and 16 but may occasionally occur earlier or later. During the first 18 months, some menstrual cycles may occur without the release of eggs. This is why periods are often erratic and of varying lengths and heaviness during the first years of adolescence.

FSH and LH hormones act on dormant egg follicles within the ovaries and switch them on. Several follicles in each ovary start to mature until one puts on a growth spurt and out-paces the rest. This is known as the dominant follicle. It is not known how or why this follicle is singled out for development, but it continues to produce increasing amounts of oestrogen. The oestrogen travels in the blood stream to the pituitary gland and damps down its secretion of FSH and LH. As a result, blood levels of FSH fall slightly. When this happens, the non-dominant follicles stop growing and regress. Only the dominant follicle continues to grow, because it has matured enough to respond to lower levels of FSH.

The Proliferative phase of the menstrual cycle

The lining of the womb responds to increasing oestrogen levels at puberty, and at the beginning of each menstrual cycle, by thickening up.

Growth of the endometrium is rapid during the first two weeks of the menstrual cycle, which is known as the proliferative (or follicular) phase. The secretory glands within the endometrium, which were short and clumpy at the end of the period, become elongated and straight as the endometrial lining thickens. By the time ovulation occurs, the endometrial lining is almost ready and waiting for implantation of a fertilised egg. During this proliferative phase, cervical mucus also becomes increasingly thin, fluid and elastic so that sperm can swim through it easily.

Ovulation

As the dominant follicle matures, the egg inside becomes suspended on a hillock in a large, fluid-filled cavity. It is now known as a Graafian follicle, after the man who first described it. After 10–14 days of growth the follicle measures 2–3 cm across and bulges from the ovary surface.

Just before ovulation, the pituitary gland secretes a flood of follicle-stimulating hormone and leutinising hormone in what is known as the LH surge. This triggers ovulation around nine hours later and the dominant follicle bursts, releasing its mature egg (ovum). Many women notice some mid-cycle pain at around this time due to the pressure within the swollen egg follicle. This pain is known as *mittelschmertz*.

As a rule, only one egg is released each month in humans. Contrary to popular belief, an egg is not released from each ovary on alternate months. There doesn't seem to be a pattern and eggs are released from the two ovaries in an irregular and unpredictable pattern.

Ovum capture

The Fallopian tubes are the site of fertilisation. They are thin-walled, muscular tubes that secrete a nourishing fluid into their lumen, or interior cavity. The inner end of each tube is open and surrounded by finger-like projections called fimbriae. The fimbriae seem to be attracted towards the developing Graafian follicle and hover around, waiting to scoop up the egg once it is released. Once ovulation occurs, the ovum is captured and directed into the Fallopian tube.

The inside surface of each Fallopian tube is covered with tiny hair-like projections (cilia) which beat rapidly to set up eddy currents. These suck the released egg into the tube and carry it downwards on the so-called ciliary escalator. Fluid currents and contraction of the muscular walls of the Fallopian tubes also help the egg's downward journey.

The Secretory phase and the corpus luteum

Up until ovulation, the endometrium has been proliferating, or thickening, under the influence of oestrogen. As soon as ovulation occurs, the empty ovarian follicle which has just released a ripe egg collapses and fills with blood. The cells surrounding the follicle, which are rich in cholesterol granules, rapidly start to proliferate. The clotted blood within the collapsed follicle is replaced with yellowish, fatty (luteal) cells to form a yellow cyst, the corpus luteum.

For around ten days after ovulation, this cyst swells until it is about 2cm across. During this time, it continues making oestrogen and also starts to secrete lots of another female hormone, progesterone. This is known as the luteal, or secretory phase of the menstrual cycle.

Progesterone has many effects. The two most important ones are:

- changing the endometrium from its oestrogen-dependent proliferative phase into the progesterone-dependent secretory phase so it can accept the fertilized egg
- preventing menstruation – thus maintaining early pregnancy should fertilisation occur.

The increasing amounts of progesterone cause blood vessels to grow rapidly into the thickened womb lining so it becomes soft, spongy, vascular and boggy.

The endometrium usually reaches a thickness of around 5mm. Its glands become coiled and tortuous and start to secrete a clear, nourishing fluid. This part of the menstrual cycle is therefore called the secretory phase. The secretions are designed to provide a fertilised egg with vital nutrients both before and after it implants.

After ovulation, cervical mucus rapidly becomes scant, thick and viscous so that sperm are unable to swim through easily.

Maintaining early pregnancy

If fertilisation occurs, the corpus luteum receives a hormone signal – human chorionic gonadotrophin (hCG) from the developing placenta of the implanted fertilised egg which keeps the corpus luteum active. After the third month of pregnancy, the placenta takes over the role of hormone production and the corpus luteum withers away. Progesterone levels remain high throughout pregnancy, and this is what prevents the womb lining from being shed. There are usually no more periods until after the baby is born.

Menstruation

If pregnancy does not occur, the corpus luteum does not receive its hCG signal. It therefore starts to degenerate around ten days after ovulation, and its production of oestrogen and progesterone rapidly tails off. This triggers menstruation around four days after the corpus luteum stops functioning. The corpus luteum (collapsed follicle) in the ovary is eventually replaced by scar tissue.

The endometrium is supplied with two types of arteries:

• The superficial two-thirds of the endometrium which is shed during menstruation (stratum functionale) is supplied by long, coiled arteries.
• The deep layer, which is not shed (stratum basale) is supplied by short, straight, basilar arteries.

During menstruation, the spiral arteries supplying the outer two-thirds of the endometrium go into spasm so the blood supply is reduced. These endometrial tissues become starved of oxygen and start to thin down and disintegrate. The top two-thirds of the endometrium is then shed and menstruation starts approximately 14 days after ovulation.

The basal layer of the endometrium continues to receive an adequate blood supply from the basilar arteries, so by the end of a period, all but the deep layers of the endometrium have been cast off.

· *Menstrual patterns* ·

The average age for the onset of menstruation (menarche) is 13.4 years, although it can occur normally at any age from 10 to 16 years. The average age when periods stop (the menopause) is 51 years.

From puberty until the menopause, women experience an average of 13 menstrual bleeds per year.

Allowing for the lack of periods occurring during pregnancy, the average modern woman will thus have between 400 and 500 periods during her life.

• By convention, the first day of bleeding is labelled day 1.
• The length of the menstrual cycle is variable. The 28-day cycle usually quoted as the average occurs in only about 12 per cent of women. Between 21 and 35 days is considered normal; however, in some women it lasts 15 days or less; in others, as many as 50 days.

- A period may last from 1 to 8 days, with 3–5 days being usual.
- The only constant factor in the cycle is that ovulation (if it does occur) takes place 14 days (plus or minus one) before the next period starts.
- By the end of a period, blood levels of the two ovarian hormones, oestrogen and progesterone, are at their lowest. This triggers production of GnRH, FSH and LH to start the next menstrual cycle.

· *Menstrual fluid* ·

Menstrual fluid contains many substances, including red blood cells, tissue debris from the womb lining, live endometrial cells, cervical mucus, sloughed vaginal cells, hormones, hormone-like substances called prostaglandins, and enzymes. The fluid lost in a normal period varies between 30 ml and 75 ml. The heaviness of a period depends on a number of factors:

- the thickness of the endometrium
- the presence of fibroids
- the presence of endometrial disease, such as adenomyosis
- the method of contraception used
- drugs taken
- blood clotting disorders.

The menstrual blood loss is mainly from arteries, with only 25 per cent coming from veins. Arterial blood, which contains oxygen from the lungs, is bright red, whereas venous blood, which is low in oxygen, is a dark purple. Young, childless women tend to describe their menstrual flow as bright red, thin, profuse and fresh. Older women tend to experience a thicker, darker flow with dark clots and a stronger odour.

· *Cycles without ovulation* ·

In some cycles, ovulation fails to occur. This is most common during the first 18 months after periods start and again as the menopause approaches. The exact reason for these 'anovulatory' cycles is not yet understood. When ovulation fails, there is no corpus luteum to secrete the progesterone hormone necessary for the secretory phase of the menstrual cycle. Oestrogens from the ovary continue to cause growth of the endometrium, however, and the proliferative phase of the cycle carries on. Soon, the womb lining becomes so thick that it outgrows its blood supply. It then becomes starved of oxygen and starts to break down, triggering what seems like a normal, if early, menstrual bleed. The time taken for bleeding to occur is variable but is usually less than 28 days from the onset of the previous period.

4

WHO GETS ENDOMETRIOSIS?

Many studies of endometriosis have tried to isolate factors that could indicate a woman's likelihood of having the illness. The following risk factors continue to be suggested by various experts.

· *Heredity* ·

There seems to be a family link to endometriosis. This may be genetic, although some researchers believe that family predisposition is not necessarily due to genetic inheritance. It could be environmental, e.g. diet or smoking. Studies show that endometriosis is present in 7 to 10 per cent of first-degree female relatives (mother, sister, daughter) of an affected woman, and 2 per cent of second-degree female relatives (grandmother, aunt, cousin). Women with an affected first-degree relative are also more likely to have a more severe version of the disease. The pattern of inheritance seems to be passed on through the mother's family rather than through the father's.

Some researchers believe that there are two forms of endometriosis, one being due to a single, inherited gene, the other being a result of non-genetic factors, e.g. diet, environment, smoking, or the interaction of several different genes.

· *Race and class* ·

Early studies suggested that endometriosis was more common in white women than black women. It was also thought to affect women from higher social classes and was even known as the 'career woman's disease'. These myths have now been disproved. Later studies, which took into account factors such as:

- availability of health care
- access to contraception
- cultural patterns of childbearing and breastfeeding
- attitudes to menstruation and menstrual pain
- assertiveness and willingness to question diagnoses
- willingness to demand investigation of symptoms

show that this supposed racial and class bias was due to other cultural variables. In fact, it is now known that black women are just as likely to suffer from endometriosis as white women.

The only women who seem to have an increased racial predisposition to the disease are the Japanese. When other cultural, social and economic variables are excluded, Japanese women still seem to be twice as likely to suffer from endometriosis as women of other races or nationalities. The reason remains a mystery but may be geneitic.

· *Age* ·

Endometriosis is often described as a disease of the fourth decade (30–40 years) of life. The peak incidence seems to occur between the ages of 35 and 44, although it can occur at any age after menstruation has started. This may reflect a delay in diagnosis.

· *Menstruation* ·

No cases of endometriosis have occurred before puberty, and the incidence of the disease tails off as the menopause approaches. Once periods have stopped, symptoms of endometriosis usually cease too. Although endometriosis can occur without cyclical ovarian activity and ovulation, any factors that stop menstruation (such as hormone therapy or pregnancy) seem to alleviate symptoms significantly.

Studies suggest that the risk of developing endometriosis is related to the frequency and length of menstruation. Women with short cycle lengths (less than 27 days) and long periods (more than 7 days) are twice as likely to develop endometriosis as women with longer cycles and shorter periods.

· *Uterine outflow obstruction* ·

Because retrograde menstruation (see page 18) is thought to be the main mechanism by which live endometrial cells get into the pelvic cavity, any condition that encourages this is associated with an increased risk of endometriosis.

In teenagers with developmental abnormalities that obstruct the normal menstrual flow (e.g. imperforate hymen, narrow or absent cervix, absent vagina) the pressure inside the uterus is increased. This triggers retrograde menstruation, and more than three out of four teenagers with developmental uterine outflow obstruction develop endometriosis.

Some scientists have suggested that women with painful periods (dysmenorrhoea) have an increased risk of developing endometriosis in the future. This may be because painful periods result from the action of hormone-like chemicals called prostaglandins. These trigger spasm within the female tract and therefore may increase the pressure inside the womb. This causes a degree of outflow obstruction and increases the regurgitation of menstrual debris through the Fallopian tubes.

This theory is supported by findings in women who have not had a child. In women who have given birth, however, there seems to be no link between painful periods and the presence of endometriosis. One suggestion is that the outflow tract is permanently dilated during childbirth, so that the spasm occurring in dysmenorrhoea is unlikely to cause an obstruction and retrograde menstruation.

Other researchers do not believe that painful periods are a risk factor for endometriosis; extensive disease has been found in women who have never had a period. Research suggests that the type of painful periods that occur in endometriosis are different from painful periods occurring in women without the disease. Certainly dysmenorrhoea is a symptom that should alert a doctor to the possibility of endometriosis and allow early diagnosis.

· *Position of uterus* ·

The uterus lies in the middle of the pelvis, suspended by several ligaments. In most women it is tilted forwards (anteverted) so that the cervix points backwards. In about 20 per cent of women, however, the womb tilts backwards (retroverted) so that the cervix points forwards. This is not usually significant, although it can increase the chance of deep pain during intercourse as the ovaries are brought into the line of fire of the thrusting penis.

Some studies suggest that women with a retroverted uterus are twice as likely to have endometriosis, although other experts dispute this. The exact reason is unknown but may be related to the parts of the pelvic floor that are exposed for cells from retrograde menstruation to settle into.

· *Hormone status* ·

Endometriosis is most common in women of childbearing age, and ectopic endometrial implants respond to the female hormone cycle. Once the menopause occurs, implants usually regress, although they can be reactivated by oestrogen replacement therapy. Some studies suggest that 8 per cent of cases of endometriosis occur over the age of 50 and in menopausal women.

However, a few cases of endometriosis have occurred in women without normal, cyclic ovarian function, such as women who have never had a period and women with polycystic ovary disease.

Confusingly, cases of active, painful endometriosis in post-menopausal women have also been described, even where there was no evidence of oestrogen activity. In one case, endometriosis was diagnosed four years after the pelvic reproductive organs (ovaries, uterus and Fallopian tubes) were removed.

A possible explanation is that after the menopause the adrenal glands continue to produce low levels of sex hormones. These tend to be masculinising hormones (one reason why women get more facial hair after the menopause) but can be converted into oestrogen by fatty (adipose) tissue. In obese women, large stores of fat may produce enough oestrogen to stop their ectopic endometrial tissue from regressing or (rarely) to trigger the disease for the first time.

The exact role of hormones in maintaining endometrial implants is still not fully understood.

· *Delayed motherhood* ·

Pregnancy is known to protect against endometriosis, and delayed motherhood (either by choice or through subfertility of either the woman or her partner) has been suggested as a risk factor for developing endometriosis. The problem with this theory is that endometriosis itself is also associated with subfertility, and the delayed childbearing may be a result of the disease rather than a possible cause, or risk factor. Theories on why pregnancy is protective include:

● exposure to high levels of oestrogen and progesterone hormones
● irreversible enlargement and dilation of the cervix (outflow tract) during vaginal delivery
● cessation of periods for around 12 months on each occasion, so that the woman is exposed to less risk of retrograde menstruation.

The jury is still out as to which factors are most important.

· *Stress* ·

It is sometimes said that endometriosis is linked to stress. Stress is known to depress the immune system – an observation that was recently strengthened when a substance secreted by nerve endings in the skin during stress (calcitonin gene-related peptide – CGRP) was discovered to damp down the immunological action of white blood cells. This provides an explanation for a link between stress, the nervous system and immune dysfunction in the skin (e.g. eczema) and it is thought that a similar substance may play a role elsewhere in the body.

As yet, the role of stress and immune dysfunction in endometriosis is poorly understood (see page 21). Although stress itself is probably not a cause of endometriosis, the pain and discomfort of the disease are certainly stressful in their own right.

· *The Oral contraceptive pill* ·

Early versions of the oral contraceptive pill (OCP) containing more than 50mcg of oestrogen may have increased the risk of developing endometriosis.

Modern formulations of the Pill, especially those containing high levels of progestogen, are used to treat endometriosis, and it is now thought that modern formulations actually protect against the disease. In one study, only 13 per cent of women with proven endometriosis had taken the OCP in the two years before diagnosis, while 87 per cent of sufferers had no exposure to possibly protective OCP hormones.

At what age does endometriosis develop?

In a survey conducted by the Endometriosis Society, 726 women with endometriosis were asked at what age they think they first started to develop symptoms; what age they were when their symptoms first prompted them to go to the doctor; and at what age their diagnosis was eventually confirmed. The results were as follows:

Age	Age when they think first began to suffer	Age when first saw GP	Age when first diagnosed
10–15	14%	5%	–
16–20	21%	10%	2%
21–25	19%	25%	21%
26–30	17%	27%	29%
31–35	9%	17%	25%
36–40	5%	10%	15%
41–45	1%	3%	5%
46–50	–	1%	2%

5

WHAT CAUSES
ENDOMETRIOSIS?

Since the early 1980s, there has been much scientific and clinical research into the possible causes of endometriosis. Despite this intense interest, however, there is still much confusion and even mystery about its origins. It is not known, for example, whether the cells that develop into ectopic endometrium become displaced before birth and lie dormant until a woman's menstrual cycle starts or whether the cells become displaced during adult life.

There are only two tissues in a woman's body from which ectopic endometrial cells could originate:

- the lining of the womb (endometrium)
- the cells that form the membrane lining of the abdominal cavity.

Various experiments have compared the surface cell receptors of these tissues, and the way they produce different chemicals, with cells found in endometriosis. Researchers have concluded that the ectopic tissue found in endometriosis is most likely to have originated from the womb. If this is the case, we then have to wonder how they get from the womb, where they are supposed to be, to other sites in the body.

· *Popular theories* ·

Ever since endometriosis was first described in the mid-1800s, various theories have been put forward in an attempt to explain its cause. Some of these theories are still popular, even though there is little scientific evidence to back them up.

Coelomic metaplasia theory

This was the first theory to be suggested, almost 100 years ago. It rests on the fact that the whole of the reproductive tract and peritoneal membrane develop from an embryonic tissue layer known as the coelomic epithelium. According to this theory, endometriosis could result from abnormalities of these primitive cells, so that patches of endometrium form throughout the genital tract instead of just in the normal place – the lining of the womb. These patches may lie dormant in some women, but be activated for some reason to form endometriosis in other women. Alternatively, normal cells within the adult female tract may unexpectedly change into a type of cell similar to that found in the endometrium. This process of one type of cell changing into another is called metaplasia. It may be triggered by contact with displaced (transplanted) endometrial tissues.

Experiments have shown that endometrial cells within a special filter chamber can trigger some changes in surrounding tissues when implanted near the peritoneal membrane. These changed cells show some similarity to endometrial glands, but do not contain endometrial framework tissue (stroma) and do not seem to function like endometrial glands.

Embryonic cell rests theory

Some scientists believe that some female embryos develop a primitive, duplicate Mullerian duct next to the main one. This might allow cells of Mullerian origin to develop into pockets of functioning endometrium within the peritoneal cavity. These small areas of resting cells are known as rests.

Direct implantation theory

This would seem to be the most likely explanation for adenomyosis. The inner layer of endometrium cells (basal layer) extends deeper into the womb muscle (myometrium) – the continuity can be seen on microscopic examination of womb tissues.

Waste ova theory

This theory suggests that not all eggs released from the ovary are successfully caught by the Fallopian tube fimbriae (see page 5) and slip down into the pelvic cavity. Some of the cells enveloping the egg in its follicle are also shed, attached to the egg. These cells have the same embryonic origin as endometrial cells, and the theory suggests that under certain hormone conditions, these might develop into patches of ectopic endometrium.

· Transplantation theories ·

Retrograde menstruation

The uterine cavity communicates freely with the peritoneal cavity through the lumen of both Fallopian tubes. During menstruation, when the lining of the womb is shed, some live endometrial cells may be wafted upwards into the Fallopian tubes and into the pelvic cavity. This is known as retrograde (backward) menstruation. A number of experiments have supported this theory:

• Live endometrial cells have been found in the menstrual flow, and in Fallopian and peritoneal fluid.

• Endometrial cells have been experimentally implanted in the peritoneal cavity and taken root and grown.

• Endometrial cells taken from menstrual blood have been successfully transplanted into the wall of the abdominal cavity.

• Female hormones (oestrogen or progesterone) don't seem to be needed for the early stages of this process (levels of both hormones are low during a period) but are important for the long-term survival of these endometrial implants.

• Endometrial implants are most commonly found near the natural position of the ends of the Fallopian tubes.

• Gravity would be expected to affect free-floating endometrial cells within the peritoneal cavity during menstruation. Hence most endometrial implants form in the lowest part of the cavity (pelvis) and sites of implantation seem to depend on whether the womb naturally slopes forwards or backwards.

• Mobile structures within the abdominal cavity (such as the bowel) are less likely to be affected (they waft free endometrial cells away from them) than fixed structures (such as the uterosacral ligament).

• The peritoneal lining is an ideal site for implantation, as it is thin, has an excellent blood supply, and is bathed in high levels of sex hormones from the ruptured ovarian follicle during the second half of the menstrual cycle and throughout menstruation (see page 7).

• Women with lax entrances from the uterus to each Fallopian tube seem more likely to get endometriosis.

• Women with a tight or closed-off cervical canal seem more likely to get endometriosis, as retrograde menstruation is more likely to occur due to the increased pressure in the womb during a period.

How common is retrograde menstruation?

Interestingly, some degree of retrograde menstruation through the Fallopian tubes seems to occur in most women during most menstrual cycles. This was first shown in women with kidney failure who were undergoing peritoneal dialysis (fluid pumped through their peritoneal cavity to extract wastes). Out of 11 women, 9 were found to have blood in their peritoneal catheter, or in the fluid flushed from their peritoneal cavity, when they were menstruating. The two women in whom it did not occur admitted to having very scanty, infrequent periods.

In one study of women undergoing keyhole surgery during their period, 90 per cent of those with normal Fallopian tubes were found to have quite a lot of blood in their peritoneal cavity. In contrast, bloody peritoneal fluid was found in only 15 per cent of women thought to have blocked Fallopian tubes – which would be expected if retrograde menstruation were occurring via the tubes.

Researchers now suspect that retrograde menstruation occurs in most women most months, and this method of endometrial transplantation probably accounts for most cases of ectopic endometrial cells found on the outer surface of the ovaries and other pelvic or abdominal organs.

Lymphatic spread

It seems possible that live endometrial cells may pass into a lymph vessel during menstruation and flow into the lymphatic system. This may explain how endometriosis is sometimes (rarely) found within lymphatic channels and lymph nodes; the first such cases were described as far back as 1925. This route of spread may also explain the cases of endometriosis around the navel as this area is rich in lymphatic channels draining from the pelvic area.

Blood spread

It is possible that live endometrial cells can pass into the blood stream during menstruation to travel around the body. This might account for the rare findings of patches of endometrium in obscure sites with good blood supplies such as the lungs, muscles and skin. How or why endometrial cells enter the blood stream is unknown, but the rarity of endometriosis outside the abdominal cavity suggests either that transplantation of endometrial cells through the blood stream is unusual or that the cells cannot survive in the blood for very long.

Iatrogenic dissemination theory

The name of this theory simply means 'caused by a physician' (from iatro, 'physician', and genre, 'causing'). It refers to surgical gynaecological procedures in which the womb is entered, that can trigger the spread of endometrial cells. The procedures that have been linked with iatrogenic endometriosis are:

- Caesarean section
- shelling out of fibroids (myomectomy – see page 145)
- hysterotomy (opening of the womb).

Iatrogenic endometriosis is thought to be rare, as it is unusual for the lower, basal layer of the endometrium to be stirred up and freed in these procedures, and it is these basal cells, rather than cells from the upper endometrial layers, that are most likely to implant elsewhere.

6

THE POSSIBLE ROLE
OF THE IMMUNE SYSTEM

Blood and live endometrial cells seem to seep from the uterine cavity into the peritoneal cavity via the Fallopian tubes (retrograde menstruation) in at least 90 per cent of all periods (see page 18). Random, single biopsies from apparently healthy tissues in the pelvis frequently show microscopic endometrial implants when examined in the laboratory, and it is suggested that they are present in most women. What we do not know is:

- whether or not these microscopic implants are the sites where live endometrial cells flushed through during retrograde menstruation have taken root and continued to grow
- whether these microscopic implants are a result of cells changing to become endometrial cells (metaplasia – see page 17)
- why these microscopic implants develop into visible endometriotic lesions in some women and not in others
- why visible endometriotic lesions cause symptoms in some women and not in others.

Many scientists believe that the immune system plays a key role in endometriosis, either in protecting against it or perhaps in triggering it.

The healthy immune system may prevent normal body cells from implanting in an abnormal site. This is backed up by evidence that skin grafts from the patient's own body are more likely to take root near their original donor site than farther away in the body. If these skin grafts are surgically transferred into the abdominal cavity, they will be infiltrated with immune cells and destroyed, even though the cells belong to the same body.

It may be that the healthy immune system normally prevents implantation of ectopic endometrial cells that are transported out of the uterus through the Fallopian tubes or in the blood or lymphatic circulation. The development of endometriosis may therefore represent an alteration or deficiency within the immune system – perhaps one that can be passed on genetically from generation to generation.

Before looking at the various theories put forward, we need to take a quick look at the immune system and how it works – one of the most complex subjects in the whole of medicine.

· *The Immune system and how it works* ·

The immune system is designed to protect us from disease. It recognises and helps to repel foreign invaders such as bacteria or viruses, foreign proteins and transplanted foreign tissues. It also wipes out abnormal or cancerous cells at an early stage before they develop into a life-threatening illness. In order to perform these functions, the cells that make up the immune system need to recognise and differentiate between normal parts of the self, abnormal parts of the self and foreign invaders.

Each body cell therefore bears an identity tag on its surface that brands it as part of the self. When a foreign cell with different surface markers is encountered, alarm bells are immediately triggered. Similarly, if a cell is encountered that bears both a self hallmark plus foreign markers (e.g. belonging to a virus, or tumour proteins) the cell is instantly recognised as undesirable and is destroyed.

The workings of the immune system can be divided into two:

- first-line, natural or non-specific immunity – protections pro-grammed into all of us as general defences against disease
- second-line, specific (acquired) immunity – specific measures aimed against particular diseases; these measures develop once we have encountered a particular infection. This provides long-term im-munity and is the basis of vaccination programmes.

· *Cells involved in the immune response* ·

All cells involved in our immune response are derived from a common stem cell in the bone marrow. These different types of immune cells work together to fight disease. They communicate by secreting chemical alarm signals (cytokines) which quickly attract other patrolling immune cells into an area and stimulate each other into a frenzy for a swift response. The main cells involved are described below.

Macrophages

Macrophage literally means 'large eater'. These scavenger cells are present in all our tissues and fluids. Somewhat confusingly, while macrophages are in the blood stream, they are referred to as monocytes.

Macrophages can contort themselves into long, thin shapes to squeeze between body cells and hunt down unwanted tissue debris and foreign material. Macrophages help to mop up the blood secreted by areas of endometriosis and break the blood haemoglobin down into a chemical called haemosiderin. This is what gives some endometriosis its blue-black look. When a macrophage comes across an invader or an infected body cell, it quickly picks up bits of foreign protein (antigen) and races off to show these to another immune cell called a lymphocyte. This stimulates the immune system's next line of defence. Macrophages also secrete chemical alarm signals which attract and activate neutrophils and other immune cells.

Neutrophils

Around 60 per cent of circulating white blood cells in the blood stream are neutrophils. They live for only 6–20 hours but play a vital role in the body's first line of defence; their absence usually proves fatal. Neutrophils engulf and digest microorganisms and help to stop their spread. Their surface membrane has special receptors for antibodies (see page 24) and for complement (see page 25) – a series of plasma enzymes which, when activated, can punch holes in abnormal body cells, infected body cells and invading micro-organisms.

Lymphocytes

The remaining 40 per cent of the circulating white cells in the blood stream are lymphocytes. There are three different types which are recognised by the way they act, and by the proteins stuck to their surface:

- natural Killer cells (10 per cent of total)
- B lymphocytes (20 per cent of total)
- T lymphocytes (70 per cent of total lymphocytes).

Natural Killer cells (NK cells, also known as Null cells) are large lymphocytes which kill abnormal body cells even though these cells have markers identifying them as part of the self. They are important in the destruction of cancer cells and cells infected with virus. They may also play a role in destroying ectopic endometrial implants.

Natural Killer cells become super-activated when stimulated by soluble alarm signals (cytokines) released by angry macrophages. This provides an important line of defence while the more specific T and B lymphocytes power themselves up into action. Unfortunately, rather like a kamikaze, the NK cell itself usually dies during its attack.

B lymphocytes make antibodies. There are many different families or lines of B cells, each of which makes one specific antibody. They patrol the body in an inactive form known as 'B memory' cells. As soon as these come across the foreign protein against which their antibody is directed, they become activated and start to produce their single, specific antibody in large numbers. These active, bristling lymphocytes are known as 'B plasma cells'. Their activity is regulated by various T lymphocytes, which act like administrators to control, encourage or inhibit their various activities.

T lymphocytes exist in several different administrative forms:

● T helper cells interact with B lymphocytes to trigger antibody production.
● T suppressor cells bring antibody production to a halt (for example, when the infection is beaten).
● T cytotoxic (killer) cells are more sophisticated versions of the natural killer (NK) cell which are allowed to attack normal body cells if necessary. These T cytotoxic cells are like professional assassins – they tend to survive their attack and go on to kill other targets.
● T hypersensitivity cells are involved in the cell-mediated, delayed hypersensitivity reactions that are linked with allergic reactions such as eczema. Allergic reactions take more than 12 hours to develop and T cytotoxic cells may be drafted in to help as well.

Antibodies

Antibodies are also known as immunoglobulins. They are a group of glycoproteins (molecules made from sugar and protein) present throughout the body fluids. They are produced by activated B lymphocytes once they have recognised a foreign invader. Each antibody is made up of four protein chains:

● two identical heavy (long) chains
● two identical light (short) chains.

These are linked together to form a Y-shaped molecule. The open end of each Y-shaped antibody clamps onto a foreign cell or protein (antigen) and clings tightly, making the equivalent of a citizen's arrest. The tail of the antibody sticks out and waits for a cop (scavenger cell, neutrophil, natural killer cell, cytotoxic T lymphocyte or part of the complement system) to come along and finish off the job.

Autoantibodies

Sometimes the immune system malfunctions in some way. It may fail to react to a potential problem, or overreact (hypersensitivity, allergy) or aim antibodies against normal body cells. This last error sometimes occurs after an infection, where it mistakes a normal human molecule for a similar-looking foreign substance which it has been fighting. It can also happen out of the blue, when for some reason the immune system fails to realise that the bit it is attacking is itself. Antibodies aimed against part of the body are called autoantibodies.

Complement

The complement system is a series of nine circulating protective proteins (C1-C9) that stick to antigen-antibody complexes in a specific sequence. This system has an in-built amplifier which triggers an increasingly rapid response. Once the first complement protein binds to an invading organism or foreign cell, it sends out a chemical scream for help until either:

- a scavenger cell comes along and swallows everything up, complement as well, or
- the other complement proteins in the series come along and team up with it. If all nine proteins build up, an enzyme is formed that can punch a hole through a cell, effectively destroying it.

Interferons

Interferons are proteins produced as a first-line defence against viral infections. They work by preventing viruses from multiplying. There are three different types: interferons alpha and beta, which are made in significant amounts by macrophages and also by any cell infected with a virus, and interferon gamma, which is made only by lymphocytes and can be triggered both by viral stimulation and by non-specific stimuli (e.g. cytokines). Interferon gamma is also able to activate macrophages and natural killer cells.

· Teamwork in the immune system ·

When we are exposed to infection, or when our immune system detects abnormal body cells, we have several lines of defence that work together to wipe out the problem. These cooperate in two basic ways to produce innate or acquired immunity.

Non-specific (innate) immunity involves cells that do not require previous exposure to a particular infection or foreign protein to be activated:

- macrophages
- neutrophils
- natural killer cells
- complement
- interferon.

Specific (acquired) immunity involves responses that are primed during a previous exposure to a particular infection or foreign protein. These agents lie dormant, to cause an explosive protective response if the invader is encountered again (this is the basis for vaccination):

– antibody response (or humoral immunity)
– T lymphocyte-mediated response (cellular immunity).

These specific defences are adaptive responses, and depend upon a previous encounter with a foreign protein. The memory of this first encounter is carried in T and B lymphocyte memory cells which circulate in a dormant state for months, or even years. They are re-activated once they come into contact with the same organism or abnormal body cell again. During this later contact, the immune system mounts a larger, more rapid attack than the first one.

· *The Immune system and endometriosis* ·

Some experts now believe that endometriosis is an auto-immune disease – that is, one in which the immune system fails or overreacts. Various scientists have studied the immune systems in women with endometriosis and have found evidence of one or more of these factors:

- increased B lymphocyte activity
- increased number of macrophages
- increased macrophage activity and secretion of growth factors
- increased tendency, in women with endometriosis who are infertile, for macrophages to engulf normal sperm
- reduced T lymphocyte activity
- decreased activity of natural killer cells in both blood and peritoneal fluid
- decreased activity of T cytotoxic cells but only in endometrial tissue and not elsewhere in the body
- increased levels of autoantibodies aimed against endometrial and ovarian tissues (IgA and IgG) found in blood, peritoneal fluid, cervical and vaginal secretions
- increased levels of antibodies to general cell membranes
- increased numbers of B and T lymphocytes in peritoneal fluid
- increased T helper cells in peritoneal fluid and in the blood
- decreased T suppressor cells in peritoneal fluid and in the blood
- increased levels of complement and antibodies IgG in the endo-metrium, with a corresponding reduction in total complement levels.

Not all of these immune abnormalities are found in all women with endometriosis, however, so as yet there is no standard immunological test that would help to diagnose endometriosis or to pinpoint its cause.

It may be that whereas normally endometrial cells spilled into the pelvis during retrograde menstruation are mopped up and destroyed by macrophages, cytotoxic T cells, natural killer cells and T helper cells working together, in some cases, this does not occur, resulting in endometriosis. Experiments have been performed in which endometrial tissue is incubated along with immune-system cells taken from women who have endometriosis and from others who do not. The immune response is much less marked in the first group than in the second.

The Immune system, endometriosis and infertility

Although in severe cases of endometriosis extensive scarring of the Fallopian tubes may prevent sperm and egg from coming into contact, subfertility can also occur even where visible signs of the disease are minimal. In such cases an immune system malfunction linked to endometriosis may be the cause of the subfertility.

The sperm contain foreign proteins and genes. Once fertilisation has occurred, the developing embryo will bear some foreign identity tags on its surface. When the developing embryo implants in the womb, it is, in effect, acting like an organ transplant or tissue graft, which would be expected to trigger a massive immune response causing the rejection of the embryo.

In order for pregnancy to continue successfully, the immune system must naturally damp down, so that the foreign proteins (antigens) on the developing embryo are tolerated and allowed to continue to grow.

Various theories have been suggested to explain subfertility even when endometriosis seems minimal:

- abnormal ovulation, with smaller follicle size
- low levels of oestrogen and leutinising hormone
- low levels of progesterone
- inadequate luteal phase of the menstrual cycle (see page 9)
- subtle changes in basal body temperature (see page 110)
- macrophage activation and increased destruction of sperm
- soluble inflammatory agents (e.g. prostaglandins, enzymes, hydrogen peroxide) interfere with fertilisation
- increased levels of complement attract extra lymphocytes and macrophages into the area; it is possible that complement binds to sperm or egg to build up and punch a hole in them (see page 25).

Experiments have shown that peritoneal fluid from women with endometriosis does seem to inhibit binding of a sperm to an egg in the test tube. It is also less supportive of early embryo development when incubated with fertilised mouse eggs, and stops them from dividing. These findings are all thought to be related to increased macrophage activity, especially increased secretion of inflammatory chemicals.

7

ENDOMETRIAL LESIONS AND NORMAL ENDOMETRIUM

The normal endometrium contains three different types of cell:

- surface cells (epithelium)
- endometrial glands
- framework cells (stroma) which bind the glands together.

Endometriosis is most simply defined as the presence of endometrial cells outside the uterine cavity. More than 15 different types of endometrial lesion have been described. These seem to represent different stages in the evolution of the disease.

Researchers have compared the microscopic appearance of these endometrial lesions with those found in normal endometrial tissue. The ectopic implants show cyclical changes in their microscopic appearance and their enzyme content, which, although similar, are not identical to those found in the normal endometrium. For one thing, there seems to be a delay in the development of proliferative changes (in the first half of the cycle) in ectopic endometrial implants compared with normal endometrium; also, there is an incomplete secretory response during the progestational (second half) of the cycle.

It seems to be the presence of surface cells (epithelium) that decides how an area of ectopic endometrium behaves:

- When epithelium is present, the implant acts more like the superficial two-thirds of the endometrium, where secretory and blood vessel changes are associated with menstrual sloughing and bleeding
- When epithelium is absent, the ectopic endometrium seems to behave like the deeper one-third of the endometrium, which is not sloughed during menstruation.

There are three different types of peritoneal endometrial:

- Free-growing implants consisting of microscopic polyps (single or multiple) measuring around 0.5 mm across; these are usually found under a vesicle, or small sac, and are made up of endometrial framework tissues (stroma) and surface cells (epithelium); they do not contain endometrial gland openings but seem to pop up like mushrooms from a network of glandular endometrial tissue implanted beneath the peritoneum; they show cyclical secretory changes and can bleed during menstruation.

- Areas in which peritoneal cells are replaced with cells similar to the endometrial surface cells (epithelium); they may or not contain endometrial glands depending on their maturity; these are the classic lesions of peritoneal endometriosis.
- Enclosed, deeper implants in which there are endometrial glands and framework tissues (stroma) but no surface epithelial cells; cyclical changes occur only in a few cases.

In a study, around 50 per cent of endometrial lesions were found to contain epithelial cells and therefore likely to show a cyclical bleeding pattern. In lesions where there were no stroma cells, endometrial glands are enclosed in connective tissue, and these are likely to form scars.

Although these studies comparing tissues are far from complete, they will, it is hoped, identify a difference that can be used as an easy investigative and diagnostic tool in the future.

· *What lesions look like* ·

The first detailed description of the classic lesion occurring in endometriosis was published more than 100 years ago in 1893 by F.D. von Recklinghausen, the same professor of pathology after whom 'elephant man's disease' is named (neurofibromatosis). Since then, more than 15 different types of lesion have been described, based on differences in visual appearance and colour.

Atypical lesions

It was only in 1986 that the more atypical, non-haemaglobin pigment containing deposits of endometriosis was first described. This was found to have microscopic characteristics of endometrial tissue but did not have the characteristic blue or black discolouration.

They can look variously like:

- white plaques
- clear nodules
- raised, red, flame-like blisters
- yellow-brown patches
- circular defects in the peritoneum.

In one of the first studies, half the patients with symptomatic, proven endometriosis had only non-pigmented lesions. When reviewed 6–24 months later, however, many had gone on to develop typical blue-black pigmentation in previously non-pigmented, abnormal areas.

Other studies showed that around 50 per cent of women with classic coloured lesions also have non-pigmented lesions, with 13 per cent of cases having non-pigmented lesions only.

Now that atypical lesions have been recognised, more and more women are diagnosed as having endometriosis when undergoing laparoscopy to investigate infertility or pelvic pain. Previously, where the surgeon performing a laparoscopy was looking for pigmented lesions, between 10 and 15 per cent of women investigated for pelvic pain and 30–40 per cent of those with subfertility were diagnosed as having endometriosis. More recently, where women with pelvic pain and/or infertility were investigated, atypical, non-pigmented lesions were described in 70–80 per cent of cases. This suggests that at least half the cases were being under-diagnosed before and that the incidence of endometriosis may be much higher then previously thought.

The presence of atypical lesions, however, does not necessarily cause symptoms. Out of 208 healthy, fertile women undergoing laparoscopy for sterilisation, up to 22 per cent without any symptoms were found to have atypical endometrial lesions.

Microscopic lesions

To add to the confusion about how prevalent endometriosis is, and whether visually identified endometriotic lesions always represent active disease, tiny microscopic deposits of endometriosis have now been discovered in areas that look perfectly normal to the eye. A biopsy was taken randomly from healthy-looking peritoneal membrane in women with evidence of endometriosis elsewhere. Up to 25 per cent of these random samples were found to contain endometrial cells.

In another study 6 per cent of women who did not have visual evidence of endometriosis but who underwent laparoscopy for subfertility were also found to have microscopic evidence of endometrial cells when apparently healthy tissue was biopsied.

If small, random biopsies from a single site have this high a hit rate, it would suggest that larger, multiple biopsies from other normal-looking tissue in the pelvis would show a higher incidence of microscopic endometriosis. Perhaps all women are affected.

· New Diagnostic criteria needed ·

The findings mentioned above have led to some diagnostic dilemmas:

● The recognition that some women with no symptoms can have obvious, either classic or typical, endometrial deposits that are causing them no trouble means that visual inspection alone cannot be relied upon to make a diagnosis of active endometriosis.

● Similarly, the finding that microscopic deposits of endometrial cells can be found in biopsies of normal-looking tissue means that visual inspection cannot rule out endometriosis.

These findings mean that the definition of endometriosis has to be changed; otherwise the condition might be diagnosed visually during an operation in women who no longer have an active form of the disease – or excluded in those who have atypical or microscopic deposits.

Why ectopic endometrial tissue should cause a progressive, symptomatic disease in some women and not in others is a mystery. Diagnostic problems also arise if ectopic endometrial tissue is found coincidentally during other investigations – does it mean a woman has active endometriosis or not? Some experts suggest that the definition and diagnosis of endometriosis should include several different factors:

* the presence of tissue similar (when looked at under a microscope) to endometrium, found outside the uterine cavity and the uterine wall muscle (myometrium)
* which shows signs of being physiologically active
* and is associated with symptoms of local progression and destruction of surrounding tissues.

If these diagnostic pointers become widely accepted, endometriosis will not be diagnosed as often as it is at present and the incidence of the disease might seem to go down. This would be an artificial drop in the statistics due to surgeons being less ready to diagnose endometriosis as a cause of pelvic pain through a simple visual inspection of the pelvic organs. The presence of endometrial 'powder burn spots' (as the blue-black lesions are often described) may be coincidental. The visual diagnosis will need to be supported by other recognised symptoms and physical signs before it is definitely blamed for a woman's problems.

The natural progression of peritoneal lesions

Endometriosis is often described as a progressive, chronic condition with a varying number of flare-ups. However, if it were inevitably progressive, there would be many more older women with moderate or severe problems. In fact, if anything, endometriosis seems to be less common with increasing age, except perhaps around the ovaries.

Studies suggest that endometriosis is a self-limiting condition which:

* resolves spontaneously in 25 per cent of cases
* damps down and fails to deteriorate in 25 per cent of cases
* follows a slow progression from the active stage (with vesicular and nodular lesions) to an inactive stage characterised by black patches of so-called powder-burn spots in around 50 per cent of cases.

Unfortunately, researchers have not yet come up with a biochemical marker to predict which women will develop progressive disease, which will enjoy a spontaneous resolution of their symptoms and which will continue with no worsening of their problems.

Whether or not symptoms improve, regress or worsen seems to be a natural evolution of the endometriotic implants with time:

• non-pigmented, pale lesions and clear papules (little lumps) are seen in younger women – up to an average age of 21.5 years. These progress to red vesicles;

• red lesions progress to blue, black and white patches or to chocolate cyst-type lesions during the middle reproductive years;

• mature lesions progress to typical black 'powder-burn' lesions in older women;

• healing causes progression to white, fibrotic scarred areas, which sometimes become calcified, in older women.

This is supported by cases in which review laparoscopies have found classic pigmented lesions in women who previously had only atypical, non-pigmented deposits. In women followed up with regular laparoscopies, a progression from clear papules to red lesions, to classic blue and black powder-burn lesions has also been seen.

· *Activity of lesions* ·

Cells from early, or atypical, non-pigmented lesions also have more biochemical activity, when tested in the laboratory, than darker-coloured older lesions. Red implants produce twice as much of a hormone-like inflammation chemical (prostaglandin F) than brown lesions, whereas black implants don't seem to produce any at all. Other researchers have also confirmed that red implants are more active than black, puckered lesions. This decrease in activity as the lesions progress suggests a natural tendency for the disease to burn itself out.

· *Ovarian lesions* ·

The ovaries are the commonest sites where ectopic endometrial implants are found. Careful examination of ovarian endometrial cysts, shows that, in 90 per cent of cases, they form from an infolding (inversion) of the ovarian cortex. The sequence is thought to be as follows:

• These implants become connected by an extensive system of blood vessels over the surface of the ovary.

• Bleeding from ectopic endometrium triggers inflammation.

• Scar tissue forms, which contracts and pulls the ovarian cortex inwards to form a pouch.

• Mucosa-like outgrowths of ectopic endometrial tissue form on the inverted surface of the ovary.

• The inversion in the surface of the ovary becomes covered with a cap of scar tissue and forms a haemorrhagic cyst (endometrioma).

• Further bleeding into this cyst forms a pool of trapped blood and discarded endometrial tissues.

● The cyst contents break down under the action of enzymes to form a chocolate-coloured collection of material.

● Distension of the cyst and fibrosis of its wall hides its original structure and forms what looks like a bulging, dark splodge on the surface of the ovary – the classic chocolate cyst.

● If the wall of the endometrioma is thick, the cyst may look white- or yellow-tinged and can be difficult to tell apart from a corpus luteum (see page 9); the latter usually has a rupture mark (stigma) on its surface and a more vascular appearance.

Before the formation of endometriomas was understood, the condition was sometimes referred to as 'deep endometriosis'. This is now known to be misleading. The cyst forms from a combination of superficial endometriosis and scarring.

As 10 per cent of ovarian endometrial cysts do not have this architecture, it is thought that these might form when ectopic endometrial cells fall into a ruptured follicle and colonise it.

· *Malignant change* ·

Very rarely, ectopic endometrial lesions can undergo malignant change. Most cancers that arise are similar to those that can occur in normal endometrium, although a few are unusual in that they show characteristics of other types of cells.

Three-quarters of these cancers associated with endometriosis develop in endometriomas. Only one quarter are found in non-ovarian ectopic endometrial implants. Malignant changes in these ectopic endometrial lesions seem to occur ten years earlier, on average, than expected for endometrium in its normal intra-uterine site. This means that endometrioid tumours can occur in women under 40 years of age.

In 1980, doctors investigating non-ovarian ectopic endometrial cancers described 35 cases. The age range of these patients was 30 to 73, with an average age of 48. Thirteen of the ectopic endometrial cancers were in the tissue between the vagina and rectum (rectovaginal septum), four in the vagina, three in the bladder and the rest in a variety of sites including the Fallopian tubes, cervix, vulva, uterosacral ligaments, large or small bowel, umbilicus and lymph nodes.

Pain that alters in character from its usual cyclical pattern to a more constant pain is thought to be a diagnostic pointer to malignant change. If you do have this symptom, let your doctor know; but remember that these tumours are rare and that there may be no cause for alarm. Other clues that may suggest malignant change are rupture of an endometriotic ovarian cyst, and the presence of an exceptionally large endometrioma with a diameter of more than 15 cm.

8

ADENOMYOSIS

Adenomyosis is similar to endometriosis, in that ectopic endometrial deposits are found outside their normal position: in this case within the muscular wall of the womb itself, nestled between the muscle fibres.

- *adeno* means 'glands'
- *myo* means 'muscle'
- *osis* means 'disease, problem or abnormality'.

Endometrial tissue is made up of lots of endometrial secretory glands plus connective tissue (stroma) that binds them together – hence adenomyosis means a problem in which endometrial glands are found in the muscle of the womb. In older books this is often called 'internal endometriosis'.

Many experts now believe that adenomyosis is not really a form of endometriosis at all, since:

- the endometrial glands are thought to be in continuity with the endometrium and have just extended into the muscle;
- it affects women at an older age;
- it gives a different clinical pattern of problems.

Others disagree, as the endometrial cells found in adenomyosis are immature and do not seem to undergo cyclical changes like those of the endometrium.

Adenomyosis is relatively rare and can occur in two main forms:

- **diffuse adenomyosis** – in which the deposits of endometrial cells are confined to the inner part of the uterine wall, close to the womb cavity. This is the commonest type.
- **localised adenomyosis** – in which the endometrial deposits are localised to one part of the uterine wall and occur throughout its thickness, both near the cavity and close to the outer surface.

There are no specific symptoms associated with adenomyosis but many women seem to suffer pain. This may be due to swelling of the ectopic glandular cells which might push the surrounding muscle fibres apart to trigger pain. Although some of the endometrial deposits are thought to communicate with the uterine cavity, their glandular tissues often contain trapped, altered blood which also causes the glands to swell and become cystic. As this trapped blood breaks down, it sets up an inflammatory reaction which causes changes within the surrounding womb muscle. The muscle and connective (binding) tissues surrounding the area of adenomyosis tend to respond by overgrowing, to form a muscular wall that is thicker than normal.

In the diffuse type of adenomyosis, the entire muscular wall of the womb overgrows (hypertrophies) and thickens so the womb is symmetrically enlarged.

In the localised form, the muscle overgrows in one part of the uterine wall to form a solid swelling. This swelling looks and feels like a fibroid (see intra-mural fibroid, page 128) except that it is not surrounded by a capsule. Unlike a fibroid, this swelling also contains small brownish foci or pale areas with blood spots which are regions of active endometrial cells. More than one fibroid-like swelling may be present.

· *Symptoms* ·

Adenomyosis seems to be most common in women between the ages of 40 and 50, although it can occur at any age. The main symptoms include pain – especially during menstruation – and heavier periods than normal.

Adenomyosis causes heavier periods than normal in much the same way as having a fibroid does (see page 130). Thickening of the uterine wall:

- can increase the size of the womb and stretches its lining, so that there is a larger surface area of endometrium to respond to the menstrual cycle each month
- may interfere with normal contraction of the uterus and the endometrium – this contraction plays a part in closing off bleeding vessels during a period.

· *Examination findings* ·

On examination, your doctor may notice that your womb is enlarged and may be tender or feel irregular. It can be difficult, however, to tell whether you have adenomyosis or fibroids.

9

THE SYMPTOMS OF ENDOMETRIOSIS

Strangely, there is no obvious link between a woman's symptoms, how bad her endometriosis looks or how much displaced endometrial tissue is present. Symptoms seem to depend on the site of this ectopic tissue rather than on its extent. In some women, minimal signs of disease may cause maximum pain and distress. Other women with extensive, widespread disease may have no symptoms at all and be totally unaware that they are affected. Overall, it seems that 25 per cent of women with evidence of ectopic endometrial lesions have no symptoms of the disease.

Classic symptoms

The four classic symptoms of endometriosis are:

- painful periods (dysmenorrhoea)
- deep pain during sex (dyspareunia)
- pelvic pain (continuous or cyclical)
- infertility.

Other symptoms or signs that can occur include:

- heavy periods (menorrhagia)
- pelvic mass
- bowel symptoms (see page 43)
- bladder symptoms (see page 44)
- cyclical pain, swelling, bleeding or bruising elsewhere in the body (see page 45).

In general, any symptoms that are cyclical in nature, and that get worse during menstruation may be due to endometriosis.

Unfortunately, new research involving more than 2,000 women with endometriosis suggests that there is an average delay of seven years from the onset of symptoms to diagnosis of the disease. In this study, more than 80 per cent of sufferers had painful periods, 66 per cent had mid-cycle pelvic pain and 58 per cent reported pain during intercourse.

In a survey conducted by the National Endometriosis Society in 1985, 726 sufferers who experienced symptoms were asked to describe them. The results, in order of frequency, were as follows:

Symptom	% of women affected
Painful periods	94%
mild pain	6%
moderate pain	22%
severe pain	66%
Painful ovulation (mid-cycle)	77%
Swollen abdomen	77%
Loss of stale brown blood	72%
Pre-menstrual syndrome	67%
Depression	63%
Loss of large clots during a period	62%
Pain at any time	57%
Painful sex	55%
Heavy periods	48%
Painful bowel motions	48%
Constipation	45%
Nausea	42%
Back pain most of the time	42%
Back pain during periods	37%
Infertility	41%
Dizziness	33%
Difficulty sleeping due to pain	32%
Irregular periods	31%
Diarrhoea	29%
Pain on passing water	26%
Insomnia	21%
Psychological symptoms	15%
Other	13%

· *Painful periods* ·

The commonest symptom associated with endometriosis is pain. This pain is usually cyclical and linked to menstruation, although some women have pain at the time of ovulation, or throughout the menstrual cycle.

Most women notice a gradual alteration in the nature of their period pains, which alter from premenstrual discomfort to pain starting after the onset of bleeding which reaches a peak after one or two days. The pain may be felt on just one side, or on both. This progressive change in period pains is thought to reflect the progressive damage caused by active endometriosis. Once tissue damage has occurred around the endometrial implants, pelvic pain can occur outside of menstruation.

There are a number of different ways in which endometriosis can trigger menstrual pain:

- stimulation of stretch receptors (nerve endings that trigger pain) due to bleeding into a cyst (increased pressure)
- menstrual blood passing back from the womb, through the Fallopian tubes, into the abdominal cavity to irritate the sensitive peritoneal membrane lining the abdominal cavity
- the local action of hormone-like chemicals (prostaglandins) released from displaced endometrial tissues and damaged areas; prostaglandins cause spasm of blood vessels and may trigger pain through lack of oxygen in surrounding tissues
- increased cramping contraction of the womb, also triggered by prostaglandins
- irritation of sensitive bladder or bowel linings in close contact with bleeding endometriotic tissue
- increased pressure due to bleeding into the muscular wall of the uterus (adenomyosis – see page 34).

These different factors may vary in their importance in different women, or cause different levels of pain in the same woman at various times throughout her reproductive life. Painful periods are difficult to quantify objectively because pain thresholds and tolerance vary so widely from person to person and within different cultures, but the type of period pain felt during endometriosis does change over time in the majority of patients.

Many women with endometriosis have suffered with unusually painful periods ever since puberty. This may be linked with a tight cervix and outflow obstruction (see page 13). These women may feel that the quality of the period pain has not changed since the onset of endometriosis, but that the quantity has got worse.

· *Deep pain during sex* ·

Deep pain during sex (dyspareunia) is very suggestive of endometriosis. Unfortunately, it is a symptom that many women find too embarrassing to mention to their doctor. The pain may be felt only during certain sexual positions, whereas other women find intercourse impossible in any position. The causes of deep dyspareunia with endometriosis include:

- tethering of the ovaries with scar tissue so that they are in the line of fire when making love – they are just as sensitive as the male testes
- stretching of diseased uterine ligaments when the penis impinges on the cervix

- tender areas of ectopic endometrial tissue in the pouch behind the uterus which extends down between the upper vagina and rectum (pouch of Douglas)
- tender endometrial implants in the wall of tissue (septum) between the vagina and rectum
- endometrial involvement of the cervix, vagina or bladder.

· *Pelvic pain* ·

Non-specific pelvic pain can occur outside of menstruation; this is often mid-cycle, around the time of ovulation. In many cases, no obvious abnormality can be found and the cause of the pain remains uncertain. Recognised causes of pelvic pain in women with endometriosis include:

- coincidental pelvic inflammatory disease
- matting together of pelvic organs by dense adhesions which interfere with their normal movements and constrict or distort them
- symptoms resembling those of irritable bowel syndrome due to intestinal endometriosis
- distension of the ovarian follicle just before ovulation (*mittelschmertz*, or mid-cycle pain)
- distension of an ovarian cyst.

Other possible causes of pain, such as ectopic pregnancy, inflammatory bowel disease or malignancy, must obviously be considered.

· *Multiple pain symptoms* ·

Some women experience all three symptoms – painful periods (dysmenorrhoea), painful sex (dyspareunia) and pelvic pain. One study that investigated the frequency of symptom clusters found the following results:

Pain Symptom Clusters in Endometriosis

Dysmenorrhoea (dysm) only	27.9%
Dyspareunia (dysp) only	21.2%
Pelvic pain (PP) only	19.1%
Dysm + dysp	16.6%
Dysm + PP	2.3%
Dysp + PP	3.5%
Dysm + dysp + PP	9.4%

O'Connor D. T. (1987) Endometriosis. Edinburgh: Churchill Livingstone.

On investigation, it was found that women who had active endometriosis or pelvic adhesions (scar tissue) tended to suffer from deep pain during sex, pain after intercourse and recurrent pelvic or abdominal pain that was unrelated to their periods – but so do some women with a healthy-looking pelvis. There does not seem to be any significant relationship between the severity of a woman's endometriosis and the type of pain she suffers:

Type of Pain	Degree of Endometriosis		
	Mild	Moderate	Severe
Painful periods	70%	67%	44%
Painful sex	35%	41%	55%
Pain after sex	14%	17%	11%
Pelvic pain	56%	67%	55%

(Mahmood T. A. et al 1991, Menstrual symptoms in women with endometriosis; Brit J Obs Gyn 98: 558–563.

As a general rule, any woman suffering from pelvic pain or painful periods, and whose symptoms do not respond to simple painkillers such as aspirin, paracetamol or ibuprofen, may well have endometriosis and should be investigated for it. This is also true of any woman who notices cyclical symptoms such as bruising, swelling or bleeding elsewhere in the body during her period, such as bleeding from the bladder or rectum.

· *Heavy periods* ·

The average volume of menstrual fluid lost during menstruation is 30–35ml, although losses of up to 75ml are considered within normal limits.

One out of 10 women will experience heavy vaginal bleeding at some time during her life. A heavy period (menorrhagia) is officially said to occur when blood loss is greater than 80ml. However, this definition is not very helpful in practice, as one cannot very well get out the kitchen measuring spoons to measure the actual flow! As a rough guide, though, a heavy period is often accompanied by flooding and clots. Although menstrual debris contains an enzyme, fibrinogen, which breaks down clots, if the flow is heavy, the enzyme cannot cope.

If blood loss is excessive and heavy periods are allowed to continue, anaemia may result, and this can be another useful diagnostic clue.

It is not known why some women with endometriosis have heavy periods whereas others do not. Possible reasons for this include the following:

● The menorrhagia may have triggered endometriosis in the first place through increased retrograde menstruation (see page 18); studies suggest that 75 per cent of women who develop endometriosis have a history of previous heavy periods.

● Pelvic endometrial implants may cause tissue irritation, damage or scarring that interfere with normal uterine contraction during menstruation.

● Adenomyosis (endometriosis within the muscle of the uterine wall – see page 34) may interfere with contraction of the uterus; uterine contraction plays a part in constricting bleeding arteries in the unsloughed area of endometrium and helps to stop the menstrual flow.

● Coincidental disease such as fibroids or clotting disorders.

The different ways in which endometriosis pain can be controlled are covered in the Chapter 13.

· *Abnormal bleeding* ·

Between 11 and 34 per cent of women with endometriosis notice abnormal menstrual bleeding. Although the commonest type of abnormal bleeding is a heavy period (menorrhagia), the following can also occur (though they do not necessarily indicate endometriosis):

● infrequent periods (oligomenorrhoea)
● frequent periods (polymenorrhoea)
● reduction in the length of a menstrual cycle (epimenorrhoea) – that is, more frequent periods (also known as polymenorrhoea)
● premenstrual spotting of blood
● mid-cycle bleeding.

Sometimes ectopic tissues around the perineum (area between the vaginal entrance and the anus), in the vagina or on the cervix may bleed during menstruation, or when touched.

It is important to remember that abnormal bleeding from the vagina can be caused by many other conditions apart from endometriosis. Any such bleeding must be fully investigated to rule out other causes, including:

● fibroids
● endometrial polyps
● cervical polyps
● inflammation of the cervix (cervicitis)
● atypical changes in the womb lining
● pregnancy (normal or ectopic)
● miscarriage
● pelvic malignancy.

If you do suffer from abnormal periods, particularly spotting after sex, spotting mid-cycle, or bleeding after the menopause, when you thought your periods had stopped, tell your doctor straightaway.

10

ENDOMETRIOSIS OUTSIDE THE PELVIS

Ectopic endometriosis has been found in every organ system and tissue in the female body with the one exception of the spleen, which seems to be unusually resistant. A review of pathology specimens at the Johns Hopkins University Hospital, in the United States, between 1938 and 1988 failed to find one case of endometriosis involving the spleen. This fact may help future research into the cause of the disease.

Endometriosis becomes increasingly rare as the distance from the uterus and Fallopian tubes increases. Studies show widely varying figures for the number of women with endometriosis outside the pelvic cavity. Some studies suggest it occurs infrequently, in only 0.2 per cent of women, others suggest 12 per cent of sufferers are affected, while one of the largest studies, involving 2,686 women, suggests it occurred in 26.3 per cent of sufferers. Yet another study reports that 37 per cent of sufferers had bowel involvement – so there is little consensus on how common it is.

All studies agree, however, that the large intestine is the commonest site of involvement after the female reproductive organs. This would fit in with the theory of retrograde menstruation via the Fallopian tubes, which open near the appendix, lower colon and rectum. Gravity may also play a role.

Endometriosis outside the abdominal cavity is rare. When it does occur, researchers have found that 50 per cent of cases involve the lung and pleural membrane lining the chest cavity. This may be because the pleural and peritoneal membranes have a common origin (see page 6).

No single theory can explain the presence of ectopic endometrial tissue outside the abdominal cavity. Spread of cells via both the blood and lymph systems are possibilities. Whatever the mechanism, abnormalities in the immune system are likely to play a part.

For anatomical reasons, endometriosis outside the pelvis is divided into four groups:

- endometriosis involving the intestinal tract
- endometriosis involving the urinary tract
- endometriosis involving the lung and pleural cavity
- endometriosis involving other sites in the body.

· *Intestinal tract* ·

The intestines are made up of the stomach, small intestine (duodenum, ileum, jejunum), and large bowel (ascending, transverse and sigmoid colon; caecum and appendix; rectum). A large curtain of fatty tissue (omentum) hangs in front of the bowel – this contains blood vessels supplying the intestinal tract.

The incidence of endometriosis in the intestines varies in different studies, from 19 to 44 per cent of women with pelvic endometriosis.

Studies show that lesions most commonly form on the rectum or sigmoid colon, but the small intestine and appendix can be involved too. Some surgeons routinely remove the appendix when operating on women to treat endometriosis (unless surgery is for infertility, because of the additional risk of infection). It is not uncommon to find unexpected evidence of endometriosis when the appendix is examined under the microscope (between 13 and 44 per cent). Some surgeons remove the appendix only if it looks abnormal, with shortening, thickening and scarring of the wall or corkscrew deformity.

The symptoms of intestinal endometriosis (which usually occur during menstruation) include:

- abdominal pain (which may be continuous)
- distension and bloating
- constipation
- pain on defecation
- diarrhoea
- back pain
- rectal pain or spasm (tenesmus)
- rectal bleeding
- symptoms similar to irritable bowel syndrome.

Generally, the ectopic endometrial lesions are confined to the outer surface of the bowel and form small nodules. They can also be found within the bowel wall itself, or on the inner lining (mucosa).

Occasionally, the endometriosis encircles the bowel to form a ring (stricture) that can narrow the bowel. Some advanced lesions extend through the full thickness of the bowel wall, to form strictures or polyp-like masses.

Another complication is that in which loops of bowel become matted together with scar tissue (adhesions).

Strictures, masses and adhesions can all result in intestinal obstruction. Blockage of the bowel produces symptoms of vomiting, colicky abdominal pain and inability to pass wind or bowel motions. This is a surgical emergency.

In a few cases, the abdominal cavity has swollen through collection of excess peritoneal fluid (ascites).

· *Urinary tract* ·

Endometriosis involving the urinary tract (bladder, ureters, kidneys) is less common than intestinal tract endometriosis, but more common than lesions in other sites such as the lung.

Not surprisingly, the pelvic part of the urinary tract, the bladder, is most likely to be involved. Lesions are less common in the ureters and kidneys, which are farther from the womb. A survey in Brisbane found that one out of seven women with endometriosis who were investigated had urinary tract lesions, of which 98 per cent were in the bladder and 2 per cent involving the ureters. Most women are affected on only one side, but occasionally, both left and right ureters or kidneys are involved.

Symptoms of endometriosis of the urinary tract (which usually occur during menstruation) include:

- blood in the urine (haematuria), mostly during menstruation
- pain on passing water (dysuria)
- urinary urgency
- urinary frequency
- pain in lower abdomen or flank.

Because the ureters are relatively narrow, endometriosis can cause them to become obstructed. This causes distension of the kidney on that side due to outflow obstruction of the urine it makes. Kidney failure and loss of kidney function unfortunately occurs silently (without symptoms) in a quarter of patients with ureteric obstruction.

· *Lungs and chest cavity* ·

Endometriosis affecting the lungs and chest wall is relatively rare. Where it does occur, it is more likely to affect the right lung and chest wall than the left. This has led some researchers to question whether endometrial cells enter the chest cavity through a small defect in the diaphragm, a defect that occurs more frequently on the right than on the left. In fact, in 33 per cent of cases, defects of the diaphragm are found. Other possible access routes include the blood and lymphatic circulations.

Symptoms of chest endometriosis (which usually occur during menstruation) include:

- cough
- coughing up blood (haemoptysis)
- chest pain
- collapsed lung (pneumothorax)
- blood in the chest cavity (haemothorax)
- breathlessness

● nodules or calcification – occasionally found on routine chest X-ray.

Interestingly, in one study of women with lung endometriosis who coughed up blood during menstruation, none had current pelvic endometriosis. Overall, however, around 70 per cent of women with ectopic endometrial lesions in the chest cavity had pelvic endometriosis too – and this is usually advanced.

· *Other sites* ·

Endometriosis in sites other than the pelvic, abdominal or chest cavities is rare, but it does happen. Unfortunately, these conditions are frequently mis-diagnosed. The best clue to what is happening is that symptoms are usually cyclic in nature and coincide with menstruation. However, these problems are often inappropriately put down to premenstrual syndrome.

As noted before, endometriosis has been discovered in virtually all organs and tissues in the female body with the exception of the spleen.

Most cases of endometriosis in unusual sites are diagnosed as a result of:

● feeling a lump
● cyclical pain
● cyclical swelling
● unusual bruising or bleeding during menstruation.

Although rare, cases in the following sites have been reported:

Symptom	Site of endometriosis
fits and headache	brain
weak foot and hip pain	sciatic nerve
back, buttock and leg pain plus weak foot	sciatic nerve
lump plus pain around navel	umbilicus
lump and pain in groin	inguinal canal
lump in Caesarean scar	surgical incision
pain in upper abdomen plus nausea and vomiting	liver
pain in flank	pancreas
pain and bleeding in thumb	thumb
pain and swelling of knee	knee
pain in thigh	thigh muscle
tender lump on pelvic bone	pubis
haemorrhage into eye	retina
pain in shoulder	phrenic nerve near diaphragm
bleeding mole	skin

Incidence of endometriosis outside the pelvis

Site	% of women whose endometriosis involves this site
small intestine	0.2%–12%
omentum (curtain of fatty tissue containing blood supply to gut)	0.6%
abdominal wall	1.4%
vaginal wall	1.6%
cervix	1.7%–2.5%
vesico-vaginal septum (between bladder and vagina)	0.1%
rectovaginal septum (between vagina and rectum)	1.6%–2.5%
rectovaginal septum plus rectum & sigmoid colon	3.9%
rectovaginal septum plus vaginal involvement	1.8%
rectum and/or sigmoid colon	13.4%–35.5%
caecum (part of bowel bearing the appendix	0.7%
appendix	0.6%–3.9%
inguinal canal	0.8%
umbilicus	0.4%–0.8%
urinary tract	1%
femoral hernia (hernia at top of leg)	0.1%
lung and pleura	51% of women with endometriosis outside the abdomen

11

How Endometriosis is Diagnosed

Despite the fact that it is so common, endometriosis is a disease that is often missed. One study found an average delay of seven years between the onset of a woman's symptoms and its correct diagnosis.

This delay in diagnosis can be due to one or more of these factors:

- Women expect to suffer with periods and do not always report worsening problems.
- Doctors expect women to suffer with their periods and do not take symptoms seriously.
- There are no symptoms or signs that definitely suggest a diagnosis of endometriosis and nothing else.
- Symptoms are often vague and can mimic other conditions such as normal period pains, irritable bowel syndrome, cystitis, ovulation pain and pelvic inflammatory disease.
- Pain on intercourse may be mis-diagnosed as psychosexual.
- Doctors may not think to include endometriosis on their list of possible causes of a woman's symptoms.
- Waiting lists for referral to a consultant gynaecologist, and then for laparoscopic investigation, may be long.

Endometriosis is diagnosed by a combination of symptoms, physical signs on examination plus investigation (e.g. laparoscopy).

Your doctor will start by taking a medical history. You will probably be asked questions about your:

- current symptoms
- menstrual history
- sexual history – and any sexually transmissable infections
- obstetric history – or length of infertility
- past medical history
- surgical history – especially abdominal operations
- family history
- current medication
- any drug allergies
- general health – for example, bowel function, urinary symptoms, chest problems, occupation, stress levels, whether you smoke, how much alcohol you drink.

There is a classic triad of two symptoms and one sign that, if combined, should alert a doctor to a possible diagnosis of endometriosis. These are:

- pelvic pain
- pelvic mass
- infertility.

Endometriosis should also be suspected as a possible diagnosis in any woman with a history of pain (abdominal or elsewhere), whether this is during menstruation, during intercourse or unrelated to her periods (i.e. non-cyclical).

Symptoms that come and go according to the menstrual cycle are highly suggestive of the disease, but may unfortunately be put down to premenstrual syndrome or ignored as part of normal period problems.

· *It's important to talk to your doctor* ·

Surveys show that most women with severe period pains are reluctant to seek help from their GP. In one national opinion poll, 90 per cent of women questioned admitted to suffering with their periods but four out of five resorted to painkillers or self-help remedies or suffered in silence until symptoms subsided. Only 18 per cent consulted their GP.

If you have symptoms that are troubling you, it's important to tell your doctor, even if they are potentially embarrassing, such as pain on intercourse or during orgasm. Unless your doctor has all the facts at his or her fingertips, he may not consider endometriosis as a likely diagnosis.

If you feel that your symptoms are not being taken seriously or are being unfairly treated as normal or to be expected, don't be afraid to say so. One of the skills of general practice is 'waiting and seeing' whether a symptom goes away, or a patient comes back. Keep going back to your doctor if you continue to have problems, until they are sorted out.

Similarly, if your doctor says something you don't understand, or uses a long medical word without thinking, don't be afraid to ask what was meant. 'Sorry, could you explain that again' is a good phrase to keep up your sleeve.

Once endometriosis is suspected from your symptoms, the next important step in diagnosis is an examination.

· *Physical examination* ·

Your doctor will need to perform the following examinations:

- an external abdominal examination for tenderness and lumps

- an internal examination to assess your vagina, uterus and ovaries for tenderness and lumps
- an examination of the rectum to feel the uterosacral ligaments running from the uterus to the back of the pelvis (sacrum) and to feel for tenderness and lumps behind the uterus.

Your doctor may also need to examine both the vagina and rectum at the same time to assess the tissues in between (rectovaginal septum – see page 50) or to feel the uterosacral ligaments better. When endometriosis is suspected, it can sometimes help to examine you twice, once in the middle of your cycle and again just before or during menstruation. This is because nodules are usually more prominent and tender during your period.

The physical findings on examination vary, depending on how severe your endometriosis is and where your implants are. Possible findings include:

- tenderness and/or nodules at the top of your vagina, especially behind the cervix
- uterine tenderness
- uterine enlargement
- a fixed uterus that has lost its normal mobility
- ovarian tenderness
- ovarian enlargement
- pelvic mass
- thickened, tender, nodular uterosacral ligaments
- nodules in the tissue between your vagina and rectum.

In some cases the examination result will be totally normal with no clues.

· *Some signs of endometriosis* ·

Tenderness

Active endometrial tissues may be swollen and engorged before menstruation. They may be surrounded by inflamed tissues that have been damaged by cyclical shedding of dying endometrial tissues and the enzymes they contain, or be matted together by scar tissues. All of these can cause tenderness and swelling.

Uterine enlargement

The uterus may be tender and enlarged, even though the site of endometriosis does not seem to involve uterine tissue. The reason for this is not yet understood. The womb can also be enlarged because of the presence of adenomyosis, or the coincidental presence of fibroids (see page 132).

Fixed, relatively immobile womb

A normal, healthy womb is usually fairly mobile and can be moved during an internal examination by gently pushing the cervix forwards or backwards. It usually tends to tilt forwards, especially in women who have not yet had children.

One of the signs that endometriosis might be present is that the womb becomes relatively immobile. It is fixed in place by the inflammation and scar tissue and may be tethered in a forward or backward angle. Most commonly, the uterus is tilted backwards by scar tissue.

Tenderness or nodules at the top of the vagina

In the space that lies behind the uterus, between it and the rectum, there is a small space known as the pouch of Douglas, after the person who discovered it. Ectopic endometrial cells in the abdominal cavity often settle here due to the downward pull of gravity. If tenderness or nodules are felt in the pouch of Douglas during an internal examination, this is a good sign that endometriosis is present. These may be most easily felt by examining the vagina and rectum at the same time. This bimanual examination can also detect areas of endometriosis in the septum between the vagina and rectum.

Tender pelvic ligaments

The womb and ovaries are held in place by several tough ligaments. During an internal examination, the utero-sacral ligaments which run from the womb to the back of the pelvis (sacrum) can sometimes be felt; these resemble large, smooth, slippery strips of pasta. If these are seeded with ectopic endometriotic cells, the ligaments may be tender or feel nodular on examination.

Ovarian involvement

It is possible to assess the ovaries by feeling the abdomen while performing a vaginal examination, and gently trying to trap an ovary between both hands. This is not always easy, especially if the ovaries are tethered in an unusual position with scar tissue – or if the doctor has very short fingers. If an ovary is seeded with endometrial implants, it may feel larger than normal or be unusually tender. In more advanced cases, an ovary may feel indented as its surface cortex becomes hardened during formation of an endometrioma (see page 32). At a later stage, the ovarian cyst may reach a size as large as 15cm in diameter and thus be easily felt by the doctor.

Pelvic mass

A pelvic mass effect is usually the result of a collection of endometriotic tissue. In advanced disease, the reproductive organs and intestines may be matted together with scar tissue. This can also be detected as a pelvic mass, which may or may not be tender.

· *Further investigations* ·

A tentative diagnosis of endometriosis can be made based on the above symptoms and findings. Before laparoscopy was available, and before minimal disease or atypical lesions were recognised as producing symptoms of endometriosis, experienced doctors who diagnosed the disease were found to have an 85 per cent accuracy rate when open abdominal operation was subsequently performed. Now that atypical lesions are recognised (see page 29) the percentage of correct diagnoses is probably closer to 100 per cent.

Unfortunately, there are still no definitive diagnostic tests for endometriosis apart from laparoscopy, biopsy and microscopy.

A patient suspected of having endometriosis may be given one or more of these screening tests:

Urinary tests

- Urinalysis – dip stick test for protein, glucose and blood cells to exclude infection, kidney problems and diabetes; if the urinary tract is involved in endometriosis, protein and blood may show positive, but this may be misinterpreted as due to an infection or kidney stones.
- Urine microscopy – for evidence of sloughed cells; may prove positive in active urinary endometriosis.
- Urine culture – for evidence of bacterial growth in urinary tract infection.

Blood tests

- Full blood count – to look for evidence of infection (raised white cell count) or anaemia (low haemoglobin concentration)
- Blood stickiness tests: erythrocyte sedimentation rate (ESR) and plasma viscosity (PV); high results are general indicators of

inflammation or disease somewhere in the body. These are likely to be normal or only slightly raised in endometriosis.

- Kidney function tests (KFTs): to measure the concentration of urea and salts (electrolytes) in the blood. If the urinary system is involved in endometriosis, these may show unexpected signs of kidney problems.
- Liver function tests (LFTs). These are unlikely to be abnormal in endometriosis but are often done as a general screen in a patient with abdominal symptoms.

Imaging techniques

Radiography Tests involving X-rays are not very helpful in the diagnosis of endometriosis. In the past, blockages of the Fallopian tubes were sometimes assessed by blowing a special dye into the womb and tubes which showed up on X-rays.

Ultrasonography Ultrasound is a painless procedure in which high-frequency sound waves are passed through your body. These bounce back off different tissue planes and are interpreted by a computer to give an image of your pelvic organs. The doctor will move a probe up and down over your abdomen. The only thing you will feel is the gooiness of the gel used to lubricate the probe – and probably the coldness of the probe. You will need to have a full bladder when this procedure is done to help with orientation of the images produced.

Occasionally, an ultrasound is done using a special probe inserted into the vagina for clearer views of certain areas.

The use of ultrasound to detect endometriosis is not routine. It fails to detect endometriosis in many women and also gives false positive results when other pelvic disease is present. However, some physicians find it useful to tell:

- the size, shape and location of pelvic masses
- the extent of disease
- whether the bowel or bladder is involved.

Others feel that it is not useful in the investigation of endometriosis as it cannot identify early focal implants in the peritoneum. The pelvic masses that are identified also vary from cystic, solid, polycystic (or multiple) to fluid-filled or mixed. There are no definitive indications that only endometriosis is present. Therefore, ultrasound cannot distinguish endometriosis from ovarian cysts, ovarian tumours, ruptured ectopic pregnancy, Fallopian tube cysts or even an abscess.

Ultrasound is very safe; it is used routinely in pregnancy to check the growth of a developing baby.

Computed tomography (CT scan) CT scans are not often used in the diagnosis of endometriosis. The procedure involves taking multiple X-ray views at different angles across your body. These are interpreted by computer to produce excellent cross–sectional images (slices) of the tissues being examined. CT scans are expensive and, although very useful in diagnosing some conditions, would expose you to unnecessary radiation with little benefit in endometriosis. Just as in ultrasound, endometriotic lesions do not give a characteristic appearance, and thus a CT scan is unhelpful as a diagnostic tool.

Magnetic resonance imaging (MRI) MRI does not use X-rays – it uses a strong magnetic field which aligns the body's molecules. A pulse of radio waves is then passed through the body to knock the molecules slightly out of alignment. As the molecules pop back into place, they emit a weak radio signal which is picked up and interpreted by a computer. Excellent cross-sectional or 3-D pictures of your body are obtained with MRI. It gives good contrast between normal and abnormal tissues and there are no known risks or side effects.

Unfortunately, MRI still cannot distinguish between endometriomas and other types of ovarian cyst. The intensity of the signal picked up from ectopic endometrial implants also varies from strong to weak. This is thought to relate to the amount of blood (containing iron) in lesions and whether or not they are pigmented. The ability to recognise small endometriotic implants therefore varies, depending on the capacity of the machine, but it is often able to mark out the extent of the disease.

MRI can be helpful where bowel or bladder involvement is suspected; however, because it is expensive, few doctors use MRI to investigate endometriosis.

Laparoscopy

Laparoscopy is the gold-standard investigation of choice in the diagnosis and classification of endometriosis. It is also becoming an increasingly important treatment technique (see page 89). The pelvis is not a hollow space with the reproductive organs sitting nicely exposed – it is packed with organs and fluids, and identifying even normal anatomical structures – let alone tiny endometrial lesions – can be difficult, especially if bands of scar tissue are present.

The accuracy of diagnostic laparoscopy depends on a number of factors:

- the skill of the doctor
- whether or not there is any pelvic inflammatory disease or adhesions, which can obscure the view
- your size – excess weight and internal fatty tissues can obscure the view.

You will be warned beforehand that, if necessary, the surgeon may have to proceed to an open operation (laparotomy) through a 15cm horizontal cut just above your pubic bone. This is done only if the surgeon's view is impossibly poor or if a problem needing further urgent investigation is found.

One study showed that where endometriosis is present, it is accurately diagnosed in 70 per cent of laparoscopic investigations. Where the surgeon was expecting to find it (having considered the diagnosis beforehand) accuracy improved to 90 per cent, but where the surgeon was expecting to find fibroids, ovarian cancer, ectopic pregnancy or pelvic inflammatory disease, endometriosis was picked up in only half the cases where it was present. This study suggests that pre-operative bias affects the skill of the surgeon; however, it was carried out way back in 1968 when laparoscopy was new and the evolution of endometriosis poorly understood. Today gynaecologists are more experienced in laparoscopic techniques, more aware of endometriosis as a disease, and much more likely to have considered the diagnosis. They are also more aware that minimal disease can cause symptoms, and of the occurrence of atypical lesions; so don't let this commonly quoted trial put you off.

If you wonder whether your symptoms are due to endometriosis, however, and your doctor/gynaecologist has not raised this possibility with you, make sure you ask all the questions that worry you before the investigation takes place.

During the laparoscopy, your pelvis is examined systematically to ensure that no areas or lesions are missed. The most common sites for ectopic endometrial implants to lurk are (in descending order):

- an ovary – usually both are affected
- the back wall of the uterus
- the broad ligament suspending the uterus
- the uterosacral ligaments supporting the uterus
- the pouch of Douglas (behind the uterus)
- the lower (sigmoid) colon and rectum
- the round ligament suspending an ovary
- the outer surface of the bladder
- the lower ureters (running from kidney to bladder).

What happens in a laparoscopy

A diagnostic laparoscopy is usually planned on an outpatient basis. You will be given a light general anaesthetic to put you to sleep for the duration of the procedure, which usually takes less than half an hour. It is important to follow instructions about not eating or drinking for at least 12 hours before the time of the operation. Any food or drink in your stomach increases the risk of being sick during the anaesthetic, which is dangerous.

First of all, a small needle-like device is passed through your abdominal wall just below your navel. Carbon dioxide gas is pumped through this to push your coils of bowel away and to inflate the cavity. This helps to expose your womb and ovaries as much as possible.

Two small punctures are then made in your abdominal wall:

- one just beneath the navel; this is where the laparoscope (magnifying viewing device) is inserted
- one just above your pubic bone, through which other instruments (such as a probe, toothed grasper, hooked scissors, biopsy forceps, diathermy coagulator) are passed as needed.

This double-puncture technique lets the operator view your pelvic organs and manipulate them from two different angles. A few surgeons prefer a one-puncture technique and enter the abdominal cavity only via the navel.

While the surgeon is making the small abdominal punctures, the assistant inserts a probe into your vagina, through your cervix and up into the uterine cavity. This probe will be manipulated by the assistant to tilt the womb gently backwards and forwards as necessary to improve the surgeon's view.

Once the surgeon has inserted the laparoscope to start looking inside you, the first thing he or she will do is divide any adhesions present. Dividing the adhesions helps to improve the surgeon's view – and may also ease your symptoms. This is done with either a pair of hooked scissors, a heated cutting device (diathermy forceps) or a laser. The chosen implement is inserted through the lower abdominal puncture. A good view is essential for endometriosis to be diagnosed and its extent staged properly. The operating table will then be placed at a 10–30 degree angle, with your head tilted downwards. This encourages your intestines to ease apart and slither out of the pelvis up into the top of the abdominal cavity and improves the surgeon's view.

If any peritoneal fluid is present, this is gently sucked out and its colour and character noted. In endometriosis, and during menstruation, it is often stained with blood. Peritoneal washings may be sent off for microscopy if the presence of abnormal (malignant) cells is suspected.

The uterus is then gently pushed backwards, so the surgeon can see its front surface and your bladder. It is then tilted forwards – very gently, in case adhesions are connecting it to your lower colon or rectum – so its back surface and the pouch of Douglas behind it can be inspected.

The surgeon then uses a probe inserted into the lower abdominal puncture to hook the ligament suspending each ovary in the pelvis, and bring both ovaries forward into view. If a large endometrial cyst is present, this may be drained slowly. Any star-shaped ovarian scars are also punctured in case a cyst is lurking underneath. If cysts are found, the wall may be biopsied to rule out a cancer, and the peritoneal cavity will be thoroughly washed out at the end of the operation.

The surgeon then checks the ligaments suspending your uterus in the pelvis (broad ligament and uterosacral ligaments) and assesses their texture before moving on to look at your lower colon and rectum. Finally, the laparoscope is angled upwards and the surface of your liver is checked. If extensive adhesions have been found in the abdominal cavity, it is always difficult to know if they are due to endometriosis or to previous infection. If there are adhesions as far up as the surface of the liver, this suggests they are due to infection rather than to endometriosis.

During the laparoscopy, any suspicious lesions that are seen should be biopsied so that tissue can be examined under a microscope.

When the surgeon is satisfied that he or she has fully inspected your pelvic and abdominal cavities, he will remove the instruments, expel as much carbon dioxide gas as possible from the cavity, and close the two small puncture wounds with a stitch or a staple. Sometimes the stitch dissolves on its own. Otherwise, the stitch or staple is removed a few days later by the surgeon or your own GP.

After the operation

After the operation you may have some abdominal discomfort. This is usually due to the gas pumped into your abdomen to inflate it and often feels as if the pain is shooting up to your shoulder. A painkiller such as paracetamol is usually all that's needed.

You may notice some vaginal bleeding for a few days. You should use sanitary towels rather than tampons for absorbing this, to reduce the risk of infection.

Apart from that, you can resume sexual intercourse as soon as it is comfortable – unless your doctor tells you otherwise.

Very occasionally, the bowel, bladder or womb can be damaged during a laparoscopy. If this happens, you are likely to become ill with severe abdominal pain and a high temperature. If you are worried about your health in any way after a laparoscopy, always tell your doctor and ask for advice – especially if you develop any of these symptoms:

- severe or increasing pain
- fever or chills
- nausea or vomiting
- redness or swelling around your incisions
- heavy or persistent vaginal bleeding
- an unpleasant-smelling vaginal discharge
- problems passing water or opening your bowels.

Diagnostic problems with laparoscropy

Although visual inspection of the pelvic organs during laparoscopy is useful, it can be misleading, for visual evidence of endometriosis may not prove active disease is present; conversely, endometriosis can be found on microscopic analysis of tissues that look normal to the naked eye (see page 30).

Endometriosis also has several different appearances when viewed through a laparoscope. Lesions have been variously described as looking like:

- powder burn spots (dark speckles)
- brownish discoloured peritoneal membrane tissue
- bruise-like areas
- raised, red superficial nodules
- red-blue invasive nodules
- fibrous white nodules
- raised, glossy, translucent vesicles
- white, pearly, thickened patches
- red, blue or chocolate-coloured ovarian cysts
- congested superficial blood vessels.

Classically, the lesions on the peritoneum have star-shaped scarring around them which gives a puckered look. This puckering, if it is present, is diagnostic of endometriosis and helps to distinguish lesions from more serious conditions such as secondary cancers.

In lesions where bleeding into surrounding tissues has not occurred, the peritoneal implants are non-pigmented and commonly range from 1mm to 1cm in diameter.

Suspicious lesions should always be biopsied for diagnosis. Microscopic examination of ectopic endometrial implants will show if they contain endometrial glands, framework tissue (stroma) or epithelium (see page 28).

Where possible, positive findings are photographed during the laparoscopy for documentation. A detailed drawing is also made by the surgeon. This is needed for classification and staging of your disease, to see how well your treatment works, and for future comparison should you need another laparoscopy.

Investigation of bowel involvement

If your symptoms suggest that endometriosis has involved your bowel (see page 43), further specific investigations by a gastroenterologist are needed. These may include digital rectal examination, flexible sygmoidoscopy and a barium enema.

Digital rectal examination is performed by a doctor using a gloved and lubricated finger. This feels slightly odd but should not be uncomfortable. The finger is much narrower than the average bowel movement.

Digital rectal examination is important. As well as allowing assessment of the ligaments connecting the uterus to the back of your pelvis, it is a reliable way of detecting lesions in the lower rectum. These lesions are not picked up by sygmoidoscopy or barium enema.

Flexible sygmoidoscopy involves inserting a long, thin, flexible fibre-optic scope into your lower bowel via the anus. This allows the doctor to inspect the inner surface of the sigmoid colon and rectum and to biopsy any suspicious lesions. No anaesthetic is needed. You will be asked to lie on your left side with your knees drawn up and your bottom hanging over the edge of the couch. The doctor will first gently examine your rectum in case there are any obvious abnormalities low down. The sygmoidoscope is then gently inserted. Although this instrument looks long (70cm), it is narrow and flexible. You will notice an odd sensation but it should not be too uncomfortable. The doctor will pump a small amount of air into your bowel through the scope to spread your bowel walls apart gently as the instrument advances.

Normal bowel lining is a healthy pink colour with shiny, superficial blood vessels. If any unusual lesions are seen, these are biopsied with a tiny pair of pincers passed through the scope.

When the sygmoidoscope is withdrawn, the air that was pumped in will escape. Don't be embarrassed by this sound; the doctor caused it, not you, and it happens every time.

A barium enema involves filling your lower bowel with fluid introduced via a tube that is inserted through your rectum into the lower colon. The fluid is made by mixing powdered barium sulphate with water. Barium is a metallic element that shows up well on X-rays. This outlines the inner surface of your bowel and the image will detect areas of constriction, fleshy growths or irregularities of the inner bowel wall. For a single-contrast image, only barium liquid is used. This is best for showing up large lesions or constrictions. For a double-contrast image, barium liquid is introduced first, followed by some air. This means that the barium does not fill your bowel but just outlines its inner surface. This technique reveals small surface abnormalities that would not be visible using the single-contrast technique.

During the investigation, you will lie on a special tilting bed. This allows the radiologist to tilt your body if necessary so the barium outlines your bowel better. A fluorescent screen allows the radiologist to follow the progress of your investigation and to take permanent X-ray recordings or video footage when unusual areas show up. The whole procedure takes around 20 minutes and is only mildly uncomfortable.

For a successful investigation, your bowel needs to be empty. You will therefore be asked to follow a low-fibre diet for three days beforehand. You will also be given a powerful laxative to use 24 hours before; this ensures that your bowel is clean and empty. Colonic irrigation is performed just before the test.

After the examination, most of the barium fluid is drained from your bowels immediately. The rest is excreted naturally with your motions, making them thicker than usual, with a white stain.

A barium enema does not show up the lowest part of the rectum, and a rectal examination plus sygmoidoscopy will usually be done before the enema is requested.

Investigation of urinary tract involvement

If your symptoms suggest involvement of your urinary tract (pain on passing water, urinary urgency or frequency, cyclical blood staining of urine, abdominal or flank pain – see page 44) you will need other investigations including kidney function tests (see page 52), urinalysis (see page 51), cystoscopy, and intravenous urography (IVU; sometimes also called intravenous pyelography: IVP).

Cystoscopy involves a quick, light general anaesthetic. A narrow viewing device (cystoscope) similar to a laparoscope is inserted into the bladder to inspect its inner surface. Suspicious lesions can be biopsied for diagnosis.

An **IVU** involves injecting an iodine-based contrast medium into your blood stream via a vein in your arm. This substance is chosen because it shows up on X-ray, and will concentrate for a while in your kidneys as it is flushed naturally from your body. By means of a series of carefully timed X-rays taken after the injection, your kidneys, ureters and bladder can be seen in outline. If one of your ureters is blocked, the ureter and kidney above the blockage will look unusually dilated. Any irregularity of the normally smooth outline of the kidney collecting system or ureter will also show up.

Sometimes, a special compression band is placed across your abdomen for 10–20 minutes. This artificially interferes with emptying of urine into the ureters and allows the upper ureter and the kidney collecting system to dilate slightly to provide better views.

Very rarely, allergic reactions to the iodine-based contrast medium occur.

· *Diagnosing endometriosis in the future* ·

Extensive research is currently aimed at perfecting a non-invasive diagnostic test for endometriosis. This might be provided by:

- a gene
- a cell surface marker, enzyme growth factor that is present in ectopic endometrial tissue and not in normal endothelium
- a substance (such as a hormone or antibody) present in the blood in a higher or lower concentration, or in a different ratio to another substance, which is diagnostic for the presence of endometriosis
- some definite abnormality that would indicate beyond doubt that one woman has endometriosis whereas another does not
- some substance that would allow the progression of the disease, and the success of treatment, to be measured and followed.

CA–125

The best diagnostic substance found so far is a chemical dubbed CA-125, which can be measured in the blood. CA-125 is a molecule that is part protein and part sugar (glycoprotein). It is secreted by cells that are derived from developmental tissue called coelomic epithelium (see page 17). So far, CA-125 has been found on the surface of cells lining the:

- cervix
- womb
- Fallopian tubes
- chest (pleura)
- sac enclosing the heart (pericardium)

CA-125 is also abnormally secreted into surrounding fluids (from where it seeps into the blood stream) by ectopic endometrial implants and by some tumour cells. The blood test that detects levels of CA-125 is complicated and involves using special antibodies. These tests show that CA-125 is present in higher than normal amounts in the blood of:

- menstruating women
- pregnant women
- women with inflamed Fallopian tubes
- women recovering from gynaecological surgery
- some women with endometriosis
- 80 per cent of women with ovarian cancer.

It therefore is not a test that is specific for endometriosis. Tests show that abnormally high levels are present in:

- 10–70 per cent of women with mild to moderate endometriosis
- 40–100 per cent of women with moderate to severe endometriosis
- only 3 per cent of women with no evidence of endometriosis.

The sensitivity or specificity (frequency of false positives or false negatives) for this test is still uncertain. At present, its availability does not alter a woman's options in dealing with her symptoms, in that she would still need a diagnostic laparoscopy to establish whether or not she has endometriosis. However, measuring CA-125 levels may be helpful in following the course of endometriosis and the effects of different treatments.

A recent advance involved labelling antibodies to CA-125 with radioactive iodine and injecting them into two women with endometriosis. The antibodies homed in on ectopic endometrial tissue and stuck to it. Radiological imaging (scintigram) was able to pick up the small amount of radioactive signal given off by the iodine label attached to each antibody to see where the antibody had landed. In one woman, a large, 7cm ovarian endometrial cyst was clearly seen on the image. In the other case, however, the image obtained did not accurately indicate the severity of her disease. Further research is continuing into immunoscintigraphy as a possible future diagnostic technique.

Another test has found anti-endometrial antibodies in three-quarters of women with untreated endometriosis. Unfortunately, this finding is not sensitive enough to be used as a screening test, but further research into the immune side of endometriosis continues.

Laser-induced luminescence

Human tissues have a natural tendency to fluoresce. When fluorescent tissue has light shone on it, it absorbs some of the light radiation, and gives it out again as energy at a different wavelength, which can be measured by an instrument called a spectrofluorometer. Researchers in this area have investigated whether ectopic endometrial tissues could be identified by exposing it to certain wavelengths, or whether a drug could be given that would concentrate in the implants to increase their fluorescent ability (photoenhancer).

Tests in the laboratory using laser-induced fluorescence have obtained a low-intensity blue fluorescence from endometriotic implant tissues, against a bright yellow fluorescence from surrounding peritoneum. When tissues were incubated with the antibiotic tetracycline, the implants glowed with a stronger blue or blue-green colour.

Variable results have been found in clinical tests. In some cases ectopic implants that do not contain endometrial glands and those that contain a haemorrhage have failed to fluoresce. Other implants have shown up as an intense area of yellow fluorescence against the dim yellow, or white fluorescence of nearby peritoneum or ovarian tissues –but only if a chemical photoenhancer (tetracycline, or another drug, tamoxifen) was present.

These experiments have shown that the basic principle of fluorescence may be useful for identifying lesions at laparoscopy – but only if a more specific photoenhancer chemical can be found.

The search for an ideal, non-invasive, accurate, diagnostic test for endometriosis continues!

12

CLASSIFICATION OF ENDOMETRIOSIS

It is important to have a widely accepted way of classifying endometriosis so that:

- all those involved in researching and treating the disease can talk in a common language;
- each woman's disease can be carefully characterised in a standard way;
- the extent of the disease can provide a guideline for treatment;
- a woman can be given likely outcomes for future fertility, relief of pelvic pain and the chance of recurrences.

Unfortunately, the currently used method of classifying endometriosis is not perfect. A woman with mild endometriosis may have considerably more pain and problems than a woman who is diagnosed as having severe or extensive endometriosis. This is because classification is related to a woman's chance of infertility rather than to the pain and suffering she experiences. It is upsetting to be told you have mild disease when you are in constant pain and are unable to have intercourse any more.

An ideal classification which would allow a prediction of future conception, relief of pelvic pain and the risk of recurrence as well as the risk to fertility is still sought. Unfortunately, until the natural history of the disease is better understood, and the relationship between implants, pain and fertility is worked out, a perfect classification is impossible.

The American Fertility Society classification system

In 1979, the American Fertility Society published its classification system for endometriosis. This was revised in 1985 and is now widely used. The system assigns points for various features of endometriosis such as:

- site of involvement (peritoneum, right and/or left ovary, cul-de-sac (pouch of Douglas), left and/or right Fallopian tube

- number, depth and size of implants (superficial, deep; less than 1cm; 1–3cm; more than 3cm)
- ovarian cyst (endometrioma)
- the degree of adhesions (filmy, dense, obliteration of cul-de-sac; less than one-third of tube or ovary involved; more than two-thirds of tube or ovary involved).

The severity of the endometriosis is then worked out using the highest score for each lesion.

The American Fertility Society (AFS) classification is now so widely used that when discussing a patient doctors no longer refer simply to endometriosis, but refer to minimal, mild, moderate or severe endometriosis, as defined by this classification.

Although this system was drawn up by experienced surgeons, and is widely accepted, it does have drawbacks:

- Its scores are based on where visible lesions and adhesions are sited.
- The system does not take into account the cause of the disease or the extent of immune or hormonal abnormalities that might be important.
- The divisions between the minimal, mild, moderate and severe disease groups are arbitrary.
- Large variations in symptoms are seen between women with the same scores.
- Surgical expertise is needed to classify the extent of disease.

· *Expertise needed* ·

Expertise in laparoscopy is needed to classify lesions correctly. Research shows that a surgeon's ability to recognise subtle lesions increases with experience. In one recent study, the rate of patients diagnosed with subtle lesions increased fourfold (15 to 65 per cent) over two years, from 1986 to 1988, while the rate of patients with typical lesions increased by only 50 per cent (from 43 to 60 per cent) which indicates higher perception of signs rather than a higher incidence of the disease.

· *The Way forward in classification* ·

Experts are now calling for a routine description of the appearance of endometrial implants to be included in the next revision of the AFS classification, perhaps with colour pictures of atypical lesions.

Some experts also feel there is a need for an extra grade of disease – Stage V, extensive disease – perhaps for women scoring more than 70 points on the AFS classification.

The AFS is now arguing in favour of a separate classification for pain.

13

THE TREATMENT OF ENDOMETRIOSIS WITH DRUGS

If you are diagnoised as having endometriosis, the treatment will have three primary aims:

- the relief of your symptoms through surgical removal or drug resolution of active endometrial implants
- the limitation of your disease so that it does not progress, and recurrences are delayed
- the restoration of fertility, if desired.

The ultimate ideal is for you to return to a healthy, pain-free, fertile state. The choice of treatment to achieve these aims depends on several different things:

- how active and advanced your endometriosis is
- how bad your symptoms are
- whether you hope for a future pregnancy
- your age
- whether your main symptoms are pain, a pelvic mass (such as an ovarian cyst causing painful sex) or infertility.

· *Drugs versus surgery* ·

The treatment can be medical (drug treatment), surgical or a combination of the two. There are two advantages of drug treatment:

- It treats microscopic lesions not visible to the surgeon.
- It avoids the risk of post-operative adhesions.

There are several arguments in favour of surgery:

- Limited surgery can be performed during the diagnostic laparoscopy if the disease only affects small areas;
- It does not have the side effects of drugs – although operative complications can occur;
- It does not require a 3–6 month course of treatment.

Patients with endometriosis can be broadly divided into two groups: those for whom pain is the most important symptom (roughly two-thirds of patients), and those for whom infertility is the main problem (roughly one-third of patients).

In general, if your main symptom is pain the option offered is a hormonal drug treatment, as this successfully treats pain in 85 per cent of cases (but may not be permanent and does not offer a cure).

If your main problem is infertility, you may be offered surgery (for example, to remove adhesions), hormonal treatment to shrink down the implants, or a combination of both (see chapter 14). As there is a small risk of damage to the Fallopian tubes and ovaries during surgery, many doctors prefer to try medical treatments first. But your pelvic organs may already be so damaged by endometriosis that pregnancy would be impossible without prior surgery.

If you have an ovarian cyst, you will usually be offered surgery, as this is both diagnostic and therapeutic. Hormonal treatment is helpful in only 50 per cent of women with an endometrioma, and once treatment stops the cyst tends to re-form. After surgery, you will often be offered long-term hormonal treatment.

Severity of endometriosis	Generally accepted treatment
Mild	Hormonal therapy
Moderate	Hormonal therapy followed by microsurgery or laser treatment if necessary
Severe	Microsurgery or laser treatment plus hormonal therapy – with more radical surgery if necessary

Deciding on the treatment that's right for you

Every woman is different, with different lesions, differing symptoms, and a different lifestyle and needs. You should be treated as an individual, and together, you and your doctor should work out the plan of action that is best for you. For example:

• An older woman with moderate disease and bad pelvic pain might welcome a hysterectomy.
• A younger woman who wishes to have a child is more suited to drug treatment – there is a chance that her symptoms will disappear after a future pregnancy, although they may return at any time.
• A woman approaching the menopause may prefer to try drug treatment in the hope that once her periods stop, her symptoms will

disappear for good and she can avoid surgery. Symptoms may return after the menopause, however.

The aim of medical treatment in endometriosis is to suppress ovulation (and often menstruation) for six months or longer. This usually gives a significant improvement in symptoms and in many cases causes a complete regression of visible ectopic endometrial implants with a return of fertility. Different drugs have different effects in different women so you may need to have several courses of treatment until the one that suits you best is found.

It is important that no drugs be given to treat your endometriosis until the diagnosis has been confirmed through laparoscopy (or laparotomy) and until pregnancy has been excluded through a pregnancy test. This is because hormone-manipulating drugs are harmful if inadvertently given to a woman whose symptoms are due to pregnancy.

The growth and development of ectopic endometrial implants depends upon the presence of oestrogen. Various drugs have been used to reduce the amount of oestrogen in the body in an attempt to reduce the number and size of endometrial implants. These treatments include mimicking pregnancy (pseudopregnancy regime), preventing ovulation (combined oral contraceptive pills), blocking the action of progesterone (anti-gestogens) and mimicking the menopause (pseudo-menopausal drugs). Many have proved highly successful, but are unfortunately limited by the presence of side effects in some women.

· *Oestrogen* ·

High-dose oestrogens were one of the first treatments tried back in the 1940s but did not prove very helpful. Side effects when oestrogens were used alone (blood clots, nausea, vomiting, serious endometrial changes) soon led to their disuse. However, they are still used in combination with synthetic forms of progesterone. High-dose oestrogens work by helping to fool the brain into thinking a woman is pregnant.

· *Pseudopregnancy drugs* ·

Progestogens

The word *progesterone* comes from the Latin *pro* and *gestatio* – '*for pregnancy*' – indicating its two main biological effects:

- changing an oestrogen-primed (proliferative) endometrium to a secretory one in the second half of the menstrual cycle (see page 9)
- preventing shedding of the womb lining and therefore maintaining early pregnancy (see page 9).

Secretion of natural progesterone begins from the dominant follicle just before ovulation. Production increases dramatically once ovulation occurs and the follicle collapses down to form the corpus luteum. Progesterone secretion continues throughout the second half of the menstrual cycle under the control of leutinising hormone (LH) from the pituitary gland. The highest blood concentrations naturally occur on around day 21 of the cycle and then fall as the corpus luteum fails, unless pregnancy occurs. Once progesterone production stops, menstruation starts around three days later. If fertilisation occurs, the developing placenta secretes a hormone (chorionic gonadotrophin – hCG) which keeps the corpus luteum and progesterone secretion going (see page 9).

Endometriosis has long been known to improve both during and after pregnancy. When ectopic endometrial implants are inspected during a Caesarean section, they are found to be softened, to have undergone a pregnancy reaction, called decidualisation, and to have broken down in places. This is thought to be due to the effects of progesterone.

By giving extra doses of progesterone doctors wanted to trick the body into believing it was still pregnant, so this treatment was dubbed a pseudopregnancy treatment.

Unfortunately, when natural progesterone is given by mouth, it is rapidly broken down before it can produce any effects. Researchers therefore developed a series of synthetic molecules, known as progestogens, that have effects similar to those of natural progesterone, but which are active when given by mouth.

Just like natural progesterone, these synthetic hormones all cause secretory transformation of an oestrogen-primed womb lining, but this action is unusual in that it occurs too fast (accelerated glandular response). This quickly exhausts the endometrial glands so the womb lining shrinks down. The endometrium is then unsuitable for implantation of a fertilised egg; hence the use of progestogens in the contraceptive pill.

This endometrial shrinkage (atrophy) also occurs in ectopic endometrial implants, and synthetic progestogens are therefore useful in the treatment of endometriosis.

Progestogens also lower blood levels of oestrogen and leutinising hormone which may be important in relieving endometriosis, too.

Progestogens have been used to treat endometriosis since the 1960s, and have recently become popular again because of their low cost and lower risk of side effects compared with other drugs. There is little evidence that one synthetic progestogen is better than another. Those most commonly used in the UK include:

- medroxyprogesterone acetate (MPA)
- norethisterone
- dydrogesterone.

In some countries two other progestogens, lynestrenol and norethynodrel, are also licensed for use in endometriosis.

Medroxyprogesterone acetate (MPA) Medroxyprogesterone acetate comes in tablets containing 2.5mg, 5mg or 10mg of the drug. As well as being used to treat endometriosis, it is also used to treat abnormal uterine bleeding, cancer of the uterus, absent periods (amenorrhoea) and menopausal symptoms.

The dose usually given to treat endometriosis is 10mg (1 tablet) three times per day (a total of 30mg per day) starting on the first day of a period and continuing for at least 90 consecutive days (three months). It can be taken for up to six months. Occasionally, higher doses of 20mg three times per day (or more) may be needed, depending on the extent of the symptoms and disease.

The doses used can result in unpredictable menstrual bleeding. Your periods may become more regular, become irregular and infrequent, or stop altogether. Menstruation usually returns to your normal pattern within three weeks of stopping treatment.

Research suggests that MPA reduces the amount of inflammatory exudate associated with endometriosis and also reduces the white cell count in peritoneal fluid. This reduced inflammation is thought to be due to decreased retrograde menstruation.

Three recent trials have used MPA to treat proven endometriosis. In one, 35 women were given 30mg MPA for 90 days. A significant improvement was found in all cases, and recurrence occurred in only three cases.

Another study gave a higher dose of 50mg to 21 women for four months to overcome problems of breakthrough bleeding. The average endometriosis score (using the American Fertility Society classification) dropped from 18 before treatment, to just 6 after treatment. At the end of the trial:

- 88 per cent had improvement in painful periods;
- 83 per cent had improvement of painful sex;
- 88 per cent had improvement of pelvic pain;
- 100 per cent had improvement of constipation;
- 100 per cent had improvement in urinary symptoms;
- 88 per cent had improvement in pelvic tenderness;
- 67 per cent had improvement in pelvic nodularity.

Only one patient dropped out of the trial, because she could not cope with side effects (relapse of depression). In 60 per cent there was an average weight gain of 1.5kg.

A trial comparing MPA with danazol (see page 75) showed them to be equally effective, with 63 per cent of women treated with MPA enjoying a total or partial cure of their symptoms compared with 60 per cent of patients receiving danazol. Women taking MPA were more likely to have problems with fluid retention, whereas those on danazol were more likely to suffer from acne or muscle cramps.

MPA should not be taken by women who:

- are pregnant
- are breast-feeding (unless the doctor instructs otherwise)
- have hormone-dependent cancer (e.g. breast cancer)
- have undiagnosed, abnormal vaginal bleeding
- have liver problems
- are known to be sensitive to MPA.

The drug is used with caution in women with asthma, heart or kidney problems, diabetes, epilepsy or migraine, who are monitored carefully in case it makes their other problems worse.

Treatment with MPA should not start until you have had a negative pregnancy test. You should continue to use a barrier method of contraception throughout.

MPA is also available in an injectable form in which 50mg is given once a week (into a muscle), or 100mg once a fortnight. Many women, such as those who have difficulty swallowing or remembering to take tablets, prefer to take it in this form. However, injectable MPA is much more likely to cause a cessation of periods, which can be prolonged. Other possible side effects include irregular, prolonged or heavy vaginal bleeding during the first two or three menstrual cycles, back pain, weight gain and fluid retention.

Dydrogesterone This drug comes in the form of tablets containing 10 mg of the drug. It has also been used to help women with absent periods (by triggering shedding of the endometrium when the drug is stopped), painful periods, premenstrual syndrome, abnormal uterine bleeding, infertility and threatened miscarriage.

The dose usually recommended is 10mg–30mg daily for 6–12 months. It may be given continuously, or only from day 5 to day 25 of the monthly cycle. Some gynaecologists prefer to use higher doses of 30–60mg in severe endometriosis to stop menstruation altogether.

When dydrogesterone was given to 45 women with proven endometriosis at a dose of 10mg per day for nine months, it achieved complete pain relief in 89 per cent. Out of the 32 patients who later had a repeat laparoscopy, 30 were found to be cured of endometriosis. Of these, 21 had a totally normal pelvis while 9 had endometrial lesions that had regressed. None of the women suffered from breakthrough bleeding; all described their periods as regular.

Unlike other progestogens, dydrogesterone does not have a contraceptive effect and can be used in pregnancy (for example, for threatened miscarriage). In fact, there are no known conditions in which a woman should not take it.

If taking dydrogesterone you should continue to use a barrier method of contraception throughout your course of treatment, unless your doctor tells you otherwise.

Norethisterone This drug is available as 5mg tablets. As well as being used in endometriosis, it can also treat heavy, frequent periods and premenstrual syndrome and can postpone menstruation (for example, if a period is due on a holiday).

The usual dose range varies from 10mg to 25mg per day. It is generally started on the 5th day of your period (after a negative pregnancy test) and taken continuously for 4–6 months at the lowest dose necessary to stop your periods. Periods usually return within 4 to 8 weeks after treatment, although when the drug is used in short courses a period-like bleed occurs within two to three days of stopping the tablets.

In a trial in which 10–15mg norethisterone was given daily from day 5 to day 25 of the menstrual cycle, 85 per cent of women with endometriosis had significantly improved symptoms with few side effects.

Side effects are rare in doses of 15mg per day. Those that have been reported are similar to other progestogens (see below), but nausea and bloating may be more of a problem in some women.

Norethisterone should be used with caution in women with epilepsy or migraine as it may make these conditions worse.

It should not be taken by women who:

- are pregnant
- are breast-feeding
- have severe liver problems or some rare liver diseases (Dubin-Johnson and Rotor syndromes)
- have a history of jaundice in pregnancy
- have severe itching
- have a history of pemphigoid gestationis (a rare blister eruption occurring in pregnancy).

A barrier method of contraception should be used while taking this drug.

Lynestrienol In one study, 13 patients were given 5mg lynestrienol daily for nine months. The treatment was reported as successful in 90 per cent of women, with complete pain relief and shrinkage of ectopic endometrial implants. Another trial using 20 patients found that treatment failed in 8 women, however, and many reported break-through bleeding as a problem.

Trials suggest there is complete regression of endometriosis in 48 per cent of women taking lynestrienol. A quarter of women treated with lynestrienol, however, tend to have a recurrence of their symptoms within a two-year follow-up period. (NB: Lynestrienol is not licensed for use in the treatment of endometriosis in the UK.)

Norethynodrel When doses of between 40mg and 100mg per day are used, trials suggest improvement of endometriosis (with regression of implants) in 78 per cent of cases after an average of six months' treatment. Normal progestogen side effects (weight gain, nausea, fluid retention, and swollen breasts) were reported. (NB: Norethynodrel is not licensed for use in the treatment of endometriosis in the UK.)

Side effects of progestogens Very few women have to stop treatment with progestogens because of side effects. Side effects that have been reported include:

- breakthrough bleeding
- nausea
- weight gain
- fluid retention
- depression
- breast tenderness
- insomnia
- fatigue
- acne
- allergic reactions.

If very high doses of progestogens are used, extra side effects may occur. These rare problems include:

- milk production from the breasts (galactorrhoea)
- hair loss in some women (alopecia)
- excess body hair in other women (hirsuitism)
- stomach upsets (nausea, vomiting, diarrhoea)
- dry vagina.

While on treatment, you may suffer no side effects or only notice one or two; it is very rare to have more than a few. If you do notice anything that may be a side effect of the drug treatment, always tell your doctor.

Treatment with some progestogens needs to be stopped immediately if any of the following occurs:
- migrainous headaches
- unusually severe headaches
- evidence of a blood-clotting disorder
- pain or tightness in the chest
- jaundice
- general itching
- high blood pressure
- immobilisation (such as following an accident)
- the prospect of an operation within 6 weeks.

Combined oestrogen and · progestogen drugs ·

A combined preparation of oestrogen and a progestogen mimics the hormonal environment of pregnancy to stop cyclical ovarian activity and prevent ovulation.

At the same time, the endometrium (womb lining) thins down. This is the basis of the combined oral contraceptive pill, and when used as a treatment for endometriosis this is also referred to as a pseudo-pregnancy (false pregnancy) regime.

Pseudopregnancy was first used in the 1950s and was successful in relieving symptoms in some women. The doses then used were high, and over 40 per cent of women stopped treatment because of the side effects.

Modern, low-dose combined oral contraceptives have not been fully studied in the treatment of endometriosis, as other treatments such as danazol and GnRH agonists (see page 79) have been more popular.

When used for contraceptive purposes, pills are commonly taken for 21 days, and then discontinued for 7 days. During this pill-free break, the womb lining is shed. This is not really a menstrual bleed, but a physiological response to the withdrawal of the progestogen hormone. In endometriosis, a low-dose, combined oral contraceptive pill is sometimes given continuously for 4–6 months before having a pill-free break and allowing a withdrawal bleed to occur. This is effective in relieving painful periods and other pelvic pain in some women.

A trial suggested that pseudopregnancy can relieve symptoms in 30 per cent of patients, compared with a much better improvement of 86 per cent in women taking danazol (see page 75).

Pseudopregnancy is used mainly to treat endometriosis in teenagers and young women with minimal or mild disease who suffer from bad period pains. Low-dose contraceptive pills are then given for 105 days (five packs of 21 pills taken one after the other) followed by a seven-day pill-free break.

Pseudopregnancy is also sometimes used in women with recurrent ovarian cysts who may be advised to use this regime for up to five years.

· Anti-gestagen drugs ·

Gestrinone

Gestrinone is a synthetic hormone which comes in the form of a capsule containing 2.5mg of the drug. It has several different hormonal actions with some characteristics of both male and female hormones. As it does not allow early pregnancy to continue, it is classed as an antigestagen (anti-pregnancy agent).

How it works Scientists are not entirely sure how gestrinone works, but it has a number of effects that are useful in treating endometriosis. These include:

- stopping the action of an enzyme used to make hormones such as oestrogen and progesterone.
- blocking the receptors that natural progesterone binds to and reducing their number, so that the body acts as if it has no progesterone on board.
- raising the levels of active testosterone hormone in the circulation
- lowering oestrogen levels to the lower limit of normal (not post-menopausal) levels.
- lowering the average level of follicle-stimulating hormone (FSH) and preventing the mid-cycle peak.
- lowering the average level of leutinising hormone (LH) and stopping the mid-cycle LH surge which triggers ovulation around nine hours later (see page 8).

As a result of all these actions, ectopic endometrial implants degenerate when gestrinone is taken.

Dose As gestrinone lasts a long time in the body before being broken down, it needs to be taken only twice per week. The usual way to start taking it is on the first and fourth days of a period (day 1 and day 4) for the first week (after a negative pregnancy test); thereafter it is taken on the same two days of the week for the duration of treatment. The capsules come in a special calendar pack to make this easier.

The dose usually given is one capsule (2.5mg) twice per week. A recent study has also suggested that half that dose (i.e. 1.25mg twice weekly) may be just as effective and this dose may also be used in future.

Trials suggest that there is complete regression of endometriosis in 73 per cent of women taking gestrinone. The average reduction in American Fertility Score after six months of treatment with gestrinone is from 15.5 to 2. There is a rapid relief of pain, and during the first month of treatment over 60 per cent of women notice improvement or cure in symptoms of painful periods and painful sex. After four months of therapy, these symptoms improve in over 90 per cent of cases.

Gestrinone seems to be as effective as danazol and MPA. In one trial, only 17.5 per cent of women treated with gestrinone had a recurrence of their symptoms within a two-year follow-up period.

Side effects While you are taking gestrinone, ovulation is suppressed, so periods will become infrequent or stop altogether.

This is not really a side effect, but a consequence of the way gestrinone works. Depending on the dose prescribed, between 50 and 100 per cent of women stop having periods while taking it. At 2.5mg twice weekly, up to 58 per cent of women have amenorrhoea (lack of periods).

The side effects of gestrinone given as 2.5 mg twice weekly include the following:

Side effect	% of women affected
oily hair/skin	71%
acne	65%
muscle cramps	35%
breast shrinkage	29%
fluid retention	26%
itching	12%
nausea	9%
hairiness	9%
hair loss	9%
increased sex drive	9%
indigestion	3%
constipation	3%
hot flushes	3%
hoarse voice	3%
clitoral enlargement	3%

Adapted from: Coutinho EM et al, Treatment of endometriosis with gestrinone – 5 years' experience; in Medical Management of Endometriosis p 249, New York, Raven Press, 1984 (Eds Raynoud J-P et al).

Other trials have suggested weight gain in 42 per cent of women taking gestrinone.

Recently, gestrinone was given as a vaginal pessary, which seemed to produce fewer side effects and a lower weight gain while yielding the same beneficial effects.

While on treatment, you may suffer no side effects or notice only one or two – it is very rare to have more than a few. Between 52 and 89 per cent of women describe their tolerance to gestrinone as excellent or good.

If you do notice anything that may be a side effect of your drug treatment, always tell your doctor.

Women who should not take gestrinone include those who:

- are pregnant
- are breast-feeding
- have severe heart, kidney or liver failure

- have suffered from a metabolic or circulatory problem during previous oestrogen or progestogen therapy.

You must continue to use a barrier method of contraception throughout your course, until your periods return. This is usually within 18 to 36 days, with the average being 21 days after stopping treatment.

RU486 (mifepristone)

Mifepristone is a synthetic steroid hormone which has an anti-progesterone effect. It has been dubbed the 'abortion pill', as this action is used to induce therapeutic abortion within the first nine weeks of pregnancy. Because mifepristone does not allow support of early pregnancy, it is classed as an antigestagen (anti-pregnancy agent).

Mifepristone works by blocking the action of progesterone hormone in endometrial tissue. The endometrium therefore acts as if there is no progesterone present and the glands stop their secretory function and the endometrium is shed.

The use of mifepristone in endometriosis is still under investigation and it does not have a licence for this use yet. In one study involving six women on 100mg per day for three months, all noticed a significant improvement in symptoms. On repeat laparoscopy, however, there was no significant change in the extent of their disease.

Pseudomenopausal (false menopause) drugs

Danazol

Danazol is a synthetic form of the male hormone testosterone, which comes in capsules containing 100 or 200mg of the drug. As well as being used to treat endometriosis, it is also taken by women with fibrocystic breast disease, heavy periods and premenstrual syndrome.

Usually, a woman taking danazol has low oestrogen levels similar to those found after the menopause. It is therefore classed as a reversible, pseudomenopausal drug.

How it works Danazol works by producing a low-oestrogen, high-androgen (male hormone) environment in the female body. This discourages the growth of endometrial tissues and causes the endometrium and ectopic endometrial implants to shrink.

Danazol works directly on the ovaries to interfere with the enzymes responsible for the production of oestrogen and progesterone.

It also has another, indirect effect on the ovaries by working through the hypothalamus. This part of the brain is responsible for secreting a hormone called gonadotrophin releasing hormone (GnRH) which in turn kick-starts the pituitary gland to release follicle stimulating hormone (FSH) and leutinising hormone (LH – see page 8). Without FSH and LH, the ovary stops making oestrogen and eggs stop ripening. Even if FSH and LH are given artificially, danazol prevents the ovary from responding to them by blocking production of oestrogen.

Danazol also damps down some of the unwanted effects of the immune system in endometriosis. It does this by interfering with white blood cell proliferation and by suppressing the formation of antibodies directed against the endometrium (autoantibodies).

Dose Danazol treatment is usually started on the first day of a period to ensure that it is not accidentally given during pregnancy. You should also continue to use a barrier method of contraception while taking it, as it has been linked with fetal abnormalities if taken during pregnancy.

Different doctors prescribe different doses of danazol to treat endometriosis in different parts of the world. In Europe and Australia, doses of 400–600mg per day are usual, whereas in North America, doses of 800mg per day are often prescribed. Trials in which women were randomly given 100mg, 200mg, 400mg or 600mg danazol per day found:

- over 50 per cent improvement in symptoms with all doses
- no significant difference between symptom improvements with different doses
- significantly better improvements at follow-up laparoscopy among the women on higher doses
- less likelihood of a recurrence among those on higher doses.

The results also showed that the best indication of how well a woman responded to danazol was if her periods stopped and that whether or not this happened did not seem to be related to drug dosage.

The studies suggested that a minimum dose of 400mg per day was most helpful; this dose stops ovulation in over 95 per cent of women. At doses of under 200mg per day, most women continue to ovulate and only women with minimal or mild disease respond.

As a general rule, women with minimal or mild endometriosis are usually given 400mg danazol per day, whereas women with moderate or severe disease tend to receive 600–800mg per day.

Once your symptoms respond, the dose may be slowly reduced to 400mg per day. Every woman varies, however, and your doctor may decide that a different dose regime is best for you.

Most women notice a significant improvement in their symptoms within four to eight weeks of starting treatment. Comparisons between a woman's AFS score before and after treatment with danazol shows a typical reduction of 43 per cent after six months. This reduction in score is due mostly to a reduction in size and number of ectopic implants present. Unfortunately – in common with other endometriosis drugs – danazol has less effect on endometriomas (only 33 per cent resolve), and adhesions are not affected at all. For these conditions, therefore, hormonal treatment is more likely to be given after surgical correction as an adjunct.

In practice, endometriosis completely regresses in between 55 and 74 per cent of women taking 400–600mg danazol per day and some studies suggest that only 9 per cent of women have a recurrence of symptoms within two years; other researchers have found the rate to be higher.

Danazol is as effective as GnRH agonists (see page 79), MPA and gestrinone.

Periods usually return within three to eight weeks of stopping treatment.

Other uses of danazol in endometriosis Some women who are about to undergo conservative surgery for endometriosis (such as for the treatment of infertility) may be given an 8-12-week course of danazol before the operation. This makes surgery easier, by decreasing the size and number of endometrial implants to be removed, and also ensures that there are no ripe or ruptured ovarian follicles in the ovary. These would make removal of an endometrioma more difficult.

Women who are about to have a hysterectomy and removal of the ovaries (see page 152) may also be given a course of danazol before their operation. Again, this helps to reduce the size and number of ectopic endometrial implants, and by reducing inflammation, makes the surgeon's task safer and easier.

Effect on pain Over 85 per cent of women with pelvic pain notice significant relief, or cure of their symptoms when given hormonal treatment for endometriosis. Danazol has been shown to relieve:

- painful periods (dysmenorrhoea) in 75 per cent of sufferers
- painful sex (dyspareunia) in 62 per cent of sufferers
- non-cyclic pelvic pain in 59 per cent of sufferers.

When treatment is stopped, however, pain may recur within 12 months, but will usually disappear again when danazol is restarted.

Side effects of danazol Unfortunately, many women have to stop taking danazol because they are unable to put up with unwanted side effects. Three out of four women taking danazol will notice at least one unwanted effect – most of which are due to the change from a female hormone environment to a more masculine one. Most patients taking over 400mg danazol per day will stop having periods, but this is not really a side effect – it is a consequence of the way the drug works. The reported side effects of danazol include:

Side effect	% of women affected
weight gain	85%
0–1 lb	15%
1–5 lbs	22%
6–10 lbs	32%
11–15 lbs	18%
16–20 lbs	11%
shrinking breasts	48%
flushing	42%
mood change	38%
oily skin	37%
depression	32%
sweating	32%
fluid retention	28%
change in appetite	28%
acne	27%
tiredness	25%
hairiness	21%
lowered sex drive	20%
nausea	17%
headache	17%
dizziness	10%
insomnia	10%
rash	8%
increased sex drive	8%
deepening voice	7%

Adapted from the Buttran V.C. et al Interim report of a study of danazol for the treatment of endometriosis. Fertil Steril 37:478, 1982

While on treatment, you may suffer no side effects or notice only one or two; it is very rare to have them all. If you do notice anything that may be a side effect of your drug treatment, tell your doctor.

Danazol *should be stopped immediately if there is any deepening of the voice*, as this may not be reversible. In one patient, it was still present a year after treatment had stopped.

In women taking 800mg danazol per day, the average weight gain is around 4kg (8.8lb). This can be minimised by embarking on a calorie-controlled diet and an aerobic exercise programme before staring your treatment.

Danazol also has an effect on blood cholesterol levels. There are two important types of cholesterol in the circulation. One, high density HDL-cholesterol, is beneficial as it protects against coronary heart disease. This is because it is too large to seep into your artery walls and fur them up. Instead, it acts as a transport vehicle, carrying other fats around in your blood stream. The other type of cholesterol, low density LDL-cholesterol, is harmful and, if you have too much of it, increases your risk of coronary heart disease. This is because it is a small molecule that can be taken up by scavenger cells and become trapped in the artery walls. This process triggers hardening and narrowing of the arteries (atherosclerosis).

Danazol has been shown to lower the level of protective high-density HDL-cholesterol by 50 per cent and raise the level of the harmful low-density LDL-cholesterol by 40 per cent. The long-term importance of these changes is not yet known, but blood fats do return to normal within three months of stopping treatment with danazol.

Danazol should not be taken by women who:

- are pregnant
- are breast-feeding
- have porphyria (a rare metabolic disease)
- have a blood clotting disorder (thromboembolism)
- have heart, kidney or liver failure
- have male-hormone-dependent tumours
- have abnormal, undiagnosed, vaginal bleeding.

A barrier method of contraception should always be used while taking danazol.

· *GnRH agonists* ·

GnRH agonists are likely to become the most popular treatments for endometriosis in the future as they are well tolerated. They work by interfering with the action of a natural hormone, gonadotrophin-releasing hormone (GnRH).

GnRH is released in pulses every 90 minutes or so, from a part of the brain called the hypothalamus. It is a simple peptide (small protein) made up of a string of ten amino acids.

GnRH triggers secretion of follicle-stimulating hormone (FSH) and leutinising hormone (LH) from the pituitary gland, and these two hormones in turn act on the ovary to stimulate the cyclical production of oestrogen, progesterone and ripe egg follicles.

These hormones together form what is called the hypothalamo-pituitary-gonadal axis. The hypothalamus, pituitary gland and ovaries communicate with each other through the hormones they secrete into the blood stream. The oestrogen produced by the ovaries travels back to both the hypothalamus and the pituitary gland to turn them down a bit and regulate the amount of GnRH, LH and FSH they produce. The ovary also produces a hormone called inhibin, which travels back to the pituitary gland and gets it to reduce FSH production. These feedback mechanisms are clever ways of making sure the ovaries are not over-stimulated to produce too many eggs.

Scientists realised that if they could artificially reduce the amount of GnRH, FSH or LH being produced (or give large doses of oestrogen), they could treat endometriosis.

How GnRH agonists work

GnRH agonists bind to the pituitary gland at the sites (receptors) where GnRH usually triggers its action, but instead of being released in short pulses and dropping off the receptor within three and a half minutes, as GnRH does, the drugs continually bombard the pituitary gland and sit on its receptors for three to eight hours.

When the drug first binds to the pituitary receptors, it stimulates production of FSH and LH, but as it continues to sit there, the pituitary gland becomes drained and stops making both FSH and LH and GnRH receptors. It is then said to be down-regulated.

The term GnRH 'agonist' is therefore used because the drugs over-stimulate and drain the pituitary gland, rather than blocking its action as an *antagonist* would. As these drugs initially work as agonists, levels of FSH and LH start to go up for three to ten days before starting to go down. You may therefore notice a worsening of your endometriosis symptoms when you first start taking the drug. Your symptoms should start to improve after about two weeks. This is something to be ready for.

As levels of FSH and LH fall, the ovaries stop producing oestrogen, progesterone and ripe eggs and a reversible false menopause occurs. GnRH agonists are therefore classed as pseudomenopausal drugs and their effects are sometimes also described as a drug-induced, medical castration.

Unfortunately, GnRH agonists cannot be given by mouth as they are quickly broken down before they have an effect. They are therefore given either in the form of a nasal spray or by injection: under the skin (subcutaneous) or into the veins (intravenous). There are four GnRH agonists currently used to treat endometriosis:

- buserelin (a string of nine amino acids)
- goserelin (a string of ten amino acids)
- leuprorelin (a string of nine amino acids)
- nafarelin (a string of ten amino acids).

You may sometimes see the drugs referred to as GnRH *analogues*, because they closely resemble natural gonadotrophin-releasing hormone in structure. Whereas the natural GnRH peptide is made up of a string of ten amino acids, the drugs consist of a similar string (of either nine or ten amino acids) with a different amino acid in the sixth position and an absent or different amino acid in the tenth position.

Two other agonists, tryptorelin and histrelin, are also under investigation and may become available in the future.

Buserelin

Buserelin is used in the treatment of endometriosis and also for prostate cancer in men. It is available as a nasal spray or as an injection. The usual dose prescribed for endometriosis is one spray (150mcg) in each nostril, three times per day (a total of six sprays = 900mcg daily). The standard course of treatment is six months.

Treatment is started on the first or second day of your period to exclude pregnancy. If there is any doubt about whether or not you are pregnant, a negative pregnancy test is essential before your course starts.

It is best to spread the nasal sprays as evenly as possibly through each 24-hour period – e.g. early morning (8 a.m.), afternoon (2 p.m.) and late evening (8 p.m.) or similar. The effectiveness of the drug is not reduced if you have a cold, but if you have increased nasal secretions, blow your nose well before using your spray and don't use a decongestant within the 30 minutes beforehand.

In a study of 18 women with proven endometriosis, all stopped suffering any pain while taking buserelin. Of the 11 women who had previously suffered from painful periods (dysmenorrhoea) 5 were still pain-free six months after stopping treatment, 5 noticed a significant improvement and only 1 noticed no difference to the pain she had before treatment. Six of the women had pain on sex before treatment, but after three months all but one could enjoy sex with no problems.

Out of the 13 patients classified as having minimal or mild endometriosis, 12 patients had complete disappearance of visible ectopic endometrial implants at follow-up laparoscopy. The five women who were classified as having moderate or severe endometriosis had partial or complete resolution of endometrial implants, but no change in their adhesions.

Studies that compare the actions of buserelin when it is given either as a nasal spray or as a daily subcutaneous injection showed no difference in results or in side effects experienced; either formulation seems equally effective and most women would prefer the spray to a jab.

A study comparing women given buserelin as a nasal spray with women receiving it as an implant (depot of slow-release drug that needed replacement only every six weeks) found there was better suppression of the pituitary gland and ovaries, a greater improvement in laparoscopic findings and better shrinkage of endometriotic implants in the group receiving the implant. An implant is therefore under development.

During your first few weeks of treatment, you may have a period-like bleed. A few women also experience breakthrough bleeding, although this is not common. In most women periods usually resume within eight weeks of stopping treatment.

Buserelin should not be taken by women who:

- are pregnant
- are breast-feeding
- have abnormal, undiagnosed, vaginal bleeding
- have hormone-dependent cancers
- are allergic to buserelin, GnRH or benzalkonium chloride.

Women known to suffer from depression will be monitored carefully while on the treatment in case it makes their mood worse.

You should stop taking any oral contraceptive pills before or within one month of starting treatment with buserelin, and continue using a barrier method of contraception throughout your treatment. Your periods will usually return within six to eight weeks of stopping treatment.

Goserelin

Goserelin comes in the form of an injection. As well as being used in the treatment of endometriosis, it is used in the treatment of breast cancer and prostate cancer. The injection (3.6mg) contains a depot of slowly released drug which is injected under the skin on the front of the abdomen (using local anaesthetic) once a month for six months.

A recent study showed that goserelin and danazol are equally effective in treating endometriosis but that goserelin produced fewer side effects. There was a mean reduction in total American Fertility Society score of 59 per cent with goserelin and 52 per cent with danazol. Overall, 46 per cent of women on goserelin showed a clinical cure, compared with 34 per cent of women receiving danazol.

Goserelin should not be used in women who:

- are pregnant
- are breast-feeding
- are sensitive to other GnRH agonists.

It is used with caution in women with certain bone diseases.

Treatment is started only once it is certain that you are not pregnant. A barrier method of contraception should be used throughout treatment until your periods return, usually within eight weeks of stopping treatment.

Leuprorelin

Leuprorelin is used in the treatment of endometriosis and is also used to treat men with prostate cancer. It comes in the form of an injection containing 3.75mg of the drug which is usually given in the abdominal wall or thigh. Once it is injected, a constant stream of leuprorelin is slowly released over the following month. The first injection is given during the first five days of a period (after a negative pregnancy test), then given once per month for six months.

Studies comparing the use of leuprorelin with danazol to treat endometriosis show that they are equally effective, with the mean total American Fertility Society score reducing from 24 to 14 in women given leuprorelin, and from 22 to 14 in women receiving danazol.

Among the women receiving six months' treatment with leuprorelin, 99 per cent had complete cure of painful periods, 55 per cent had complete cure of pelvic pain, 64 per cent had complete resolution of pelvic tenderness and 73 per cent had a significant improvement or cure of painful sex.

Leuprorelin has also been given to women for 12 weeks before undergoing pelvic surgery and has been found to:

- reduce inflammation and blood supply around ectopic endometrial implants
- reduce the risk of adhesions after the operation
- relieve pain and other symptoms until surgery was scheduled.

Women who should not take leuprorelin include those who:

- are pregnant
- are breast-feeding
- have undiagnosed, abnormal vaginal bleeding.

Barrier methods of contraception should be used throughout treatment and until the first period returns; this usually happens within ten weeks of the final injection.

Nafarelin

Nafarelin is used only in the treatment of endometriosis. It comes in the form of a nasal spray that delivers 200mcg of active drug per spray. The recommended dose for use in endometriosis is two sprays (40mcg) per day for a total of six months. Treatment is usually started between days 2 and 4 of a period after pregnancy has been ruled out. If there is any doubt, it is started only after a negative pregnancy test.

Each spray is given to alternate nostrils, one in the morning and one in the evening.

Results in women using nafarelin are comparable with those using buserelin or danazol.

A trial in which eight women took nafarelin (400mcg twice per day) found that all had complete relief of pain. After six months' treatment, seven women had a repeat laparoscopy, in which complete disappearance of endometrial implants was found in five of them, one tiny active implant in one woman, and a persistent ovarian endometrioma in another.

Trials show that nafarelin works just as well as danazol in treating endometriosis, but with much less risk of side effects. Nafarelin also has a good effect on blood fat levels, by raising the protective HDL-cholesterol level (see pages 78–9).

Women who should not take nafarelin include those who:

● are pregnant
● are breast-feeding
● are allergic to other GnRH agonists
● have undiagnosed, abnormal vaginal bleeding

You should use a barrier method of contraception throughout your course until your periods return – usually within four to six weeks of stopping treatment.

The effectiveness of the drug is not reduced if you have a cold, but if you have increased nasal secretions, blow your nose well before using your spray and don't use a decongestant within the 30 minutes beforehand.

Side effects of GnRH agonists

Side effects of GnRH agonists are related mainly to the very low levels of oestrogen they produce in your body. Many of these (such as hot flushes) are similar to symptoms experienced by women around the time of the menopause. Possible side effects that have been reported are found on page 85.

While on treatment, you may suffer no side effects or notice only one or two; it is very rare to have them all. If you do notice anything that may be a side effect of your drug treatment, tell your doctor.

Possible long-term effects

Because GnRH agonists trigger a false (and reversible) menopause, many doctors are worried about the long-term risks of thinning bones (osteoporosis) and heart attack. Pre-menopausal women have a natural protection against these due to the effects of oestrogen on maintaining the elasticity of arterial walls and encouraging bone mineral deposition in bones.

Side effect	% of women affected (where available)			
	goserelin	buserelin	leuprorelin	nafarelin
hot flushes	98%	98%	74%	90%
sweats	67%			
acne	37%	0	11%	18%
lowered sex drive	66%	66%	13%	14%
oily hair/skin	25%			
weight gain	1%	1%	13%	–
fluid retention			5%	
nausea	5%	12%		38%
headache	59%	5%	20%	79%
hairiness	5%	0	–	2%
voice deepening	0.5%			
muscle cramps	1%			2%
vaginal dryness	75%	23%		18%
superficial pain on sex		5.2%		
breakthrough bleeding		23%		
reduced breast size	32%		2.6%	
breast pain	5%			
insomnia			17%	
mood swings	47%	10%		
nasal inflammation				18%

bruising at the site of injection
nasal irritation when given as a spray

Ovarian cysts have also been reported during the first few months of treatment (usually where polycystic ovary disease is present).

Various sources – figures for all side effects in all drugs are not available; figures also vary from trial to trial but these figures give a representative indication.

GnRH agonists do result in some bone thinning, however. Women who took 1200mcg buserelin by nasal spray per day had a 7 per cent reduction in bone density. Six months after treatment stopped, bone density was still 4 per cent lower than before treatment started. The long-term risk of developing early osteoporosis is still under investigation and for this reason treatment with GnRH agonists in women is currently limited to a single six-month course. One possible solution is to add back some oestrogen or progesterone to prevent this from happening or to combine a small dose of danazol with the GnRH agonists, as danazol helps to increase bone density slightly. As a bonus, this combination therapy involving danazol plus a GnRH agonist may have a better result in treating endometriosis, too. This treatment is being used successfully in some centres, but may not yet be widely available. Rarely, women being given GnRH agonists may enter the menopause while on treatment and will not re-start their periods once therapy stops.

Hormone effects of medical treatments in endometriosis

Drug	LH	FSH	oestrogens	androgens
combined oral contraceptives	↓ ↓	↓ ↓	↑	–
progestogens	↓	↓	↓	–
danazol	–	–	↓	↑
gestrinone	–	–	↓	↑
GnRH agonists	↓	↓	↓ ↓	↓

key

↑	= increased blood level	↓ ↓	= very decreased blood level
↓	= decreased blood level	–	= no change in blood level

· *GnRH antagonists* ·

GnRH antagonists (GnRHa) are the latest drugs under development. These work by blocking the action of natural GnRH and do not have the initial pituitary gland stimulation effect produced by the GnRH agonists. This means that low levels of oestrogen will be achieved more quickly, without the initial high that can make symptoms worse for a short period of time. Early trials involving GnRHa unfortunately found that they had unacceptable allergic side effects such as skin weals and swelling due to the release of histamine. Trials with a third generation GnRHa (antide) have shown it to be as effective and safe as danazol or GnRH agonists in the laboratory.

These drugs may become available in the future. They may well have to be used with added-back oestrogen, progestogen or danazol to protect against osteoporosis and coronary heart disease.

· *Why medical treatment sometimes fails* ·

Many studies show that drug treatment alone is often not enough to cure endometriosis. Ovarian endometriomas regress in only 30 per cent of cases after danazol therapy, and adhesions are not affected at all. Ovarian lesions greater than 1cm across in size also seem to respond less well than peritoneal implants. Results are slightly better with GnRH agonists.

When residual endometriotic lesions that have failed to regress with hormone treatment are analysed, endometrial glands are often found. Some of the cells present seem to have active cell nuclei that show continued multiplication of the cells, even when these signs are absent from cells in the normal endometrial lining. This suggests that cell division in the endometrial implants is independent of the mechanisms controlling normal endometrium. Why some residual implants do not respond to hormone therapy is not understood, but three theories are suggested:

• The drug may not be able to penetrate fully into the lesions; this is especially likely in the case of ovarian endometriomas that have a thick, fibrous (scar-tissue-like) wall.
• Ectopic endometrial cells may have their own genetic programme which overcomes the influence of hormone treatment and may continue to divide.
• Ectopic endometrial cells are more resistant to drugs as their hormone receptors may be abnormal.
• The bleeding into an ovarian endometrioma may not always come from endometrial shedding.

Twelve weeks after periods have stopped with GnRH treatment, ovarian endometrial cysts are still full of chocolate-coloured fluid. This may come from long-term oozing of blood from congested blood vessels, rather than from cyclical bleeding from ectopic endometrium. If this is the case, it is not surprising that hormonal treatment does not cause shrinkage of endometriomas in 70 per cent of cases. Other theories for the origin of this chocolate-coloured fluid include seepage of inflammatory fluid through the endometrioma cyst wall.

Some deeply infiltrating endometrial cysts have been found to contain cells with cilia on their surface similar to those found in the Fallopian tubes (see page 5). Some studies suggest these may be present in as many as 62 per cent of deeply invasive endometriomas.

As the ciliated cells found in Fallopian tubes secrete fluid into the tube to assist the passage of sperm and eggs, so, similarly, these ectopic Fallopian tube cells may be the source of some of the accumulated chocolate fluid. These cells may not respond to hormones as endometrium does, and in fact researchers have found that endometrial implants containing them are totally hormone independent.

Another problem with medical treatment is that where therapy is limited to a six-month course of treatment (for example, GnRH agonists) symptoms may eventually recur when treatment is stopped.

Whatever the cause, many women will find that their endometriosis responds better to surgery than to medical treatment.

14

THE SURGICAL TREATMENT OF ENDOMETRIOSIS

Many gynaecologists feel that surgery is one of the most exciting areas of development in the treatment of endometriosis. Modern treatments using laparoscopy and laser technology have proved successful and relatively non-invasive compared with the traditional open operation, or laparotomy. It is likely that laser treatment will become increasingly available, although the machines are expensive.

Interestingly, the act of just penetrating the abdominal cavity and pretending to do something – a sham operation – can significantly improve some patients' symptoms. These results, part of placebo-controlled clinical trials to assess treatment outcomes, are being further investigated.

There are no studies indicating the superiority of medical to surgical treatment of endometriosis, or vice versa. The decision on which treatment will suit you best is based on clinical grounds – a combination of your symptoms, signs, extent of disease, age and future plans for fertility. Surgery tends to be used where:

- an older woman's family is complete
- medical treatment fails to improve symptoms
- symptoms recur after medical treatment
- reconstruction is needed for infertility
- endometriotic cysts are causing problems
- endometriosis is extensive and severe
- adhesions are present (see page 98)
- endometriosis involves the intestines
- endometriosis involves the recto-vaginal septum
- endometriosis involves the utero-sacral ligaments
- there are peritoneal implants, especially if associated with infertility
- a woman requests it in preference to drug treatment.

If you are offered surgical treatment, the skill of the doctor and the equipment available in your local hospital will also have a bearing on the type of operation you undergo.

Many women are given a course of medical treatment before their operation, as drugs can help to reduce the inflammation and vascularity (blood supply) of implants. This makes the technical job of the surgeon easier and also seems to reduce the risk of adhesions developing after your operation (see page 99).

There are two great aims in the surgical treatment of endometriosis:

● Do no harm – care needs to be taken when using scissors or laser near essential organs; care must be taken to reduce the risk of adhesions;
● Remove as much visible endometriotic tissue as possible – this increases the chance of pain alleviation and a return to normal fertility; it also decreases the risk of recurrence in the same sites.

· *Before surgery* ·

Before a planned operation occurs, you may need to undergo further diagnostic tests (see pages 53–4) and to have your bowel emptied (see page 59).

Increasingly, patients undergoing open bowel surgery may be advised to donate two pints of their own blood in the months leading up to the planned procedure. This reduces the risks associated with transfusion if you lose too much blood during the operation. Receiving your own blood is much better than receiving someone else's!

Some surgeons also give routine antibiotics to cover the operation, so reducing the risks of infection within the abdominal cavity and subsequent adhesions and decreased fertility.

· *Conservative surgery* ·

In conservative surgery, organs, such as your womb, Fallopian tubes and ovaries, are left as intact as possible. The surgeon concentrates on removing visible endometrial implants, cysts and dividing bands of scar tissue. The two main methods are laparoscopy and laparotomy.

· *Laparoscopy* ·

Laparoscopy (see page 53) has advantages over an open operation (laparotomy) in that:

● only small incisions are needed in the abdominal wall;
● it is less likely to trigger internal adhesions;
● it is less physically invasive;
● it is cosmetically more acceptable;
● it is less intrusive to your life – you can return to work within a week.

Its disadvantage is that the surgeon needs to be experienced in examining you and wielding instruments when he or she has only a small, circular field of vision. If a laser and video camera are used, he will also have to be expert at manipulating instruments according to what he sees on the screen. This requires very special spatial awareness skills.

During a diagnostic laparoscopy, a surgeon will usually divide any adhesions he or she finds and drain any obvious endometrial cysts. If more extensive treatment is necessary, this may need to be performed during a second operation when more time can be set aside. However, many surgeons feel that diagnostic laparoscopy and laser treatment should be offered simultaneously because:

- laser vaporisation and excision of implants at diagnosis is generally beneficial;
- endometriosis may get worse before the second treatment laparoscopy can be offered;
- most women prefer to have treatment at diagnosis rather than having to wait.

Laser surgery

Laser treatment of endometriosis was first introduced as a technique during laparoscopy in 1979, although the first laser was built in 1960. It can also be used during laparotomy if appropriate.

The word 'laser' is an abbreviation for Light Amplification by Stimulated Emission of Radiation. Various gases, liquids and solids will give out light when they are stimulated by an electrical charge. The light produced by the laser is of a single wavelength (all one colour) and all the waves are in step with one another. The laser beam acts like a stream of very high-energy particles which can be projected as a parallel beam or focused very precisely onto one spot with mirrors. A small concentrated area of tissue is heated to around 2,000°F, causing the cells to explode. The precision is so great that minute burns (0.2 mm) are made with no damage to surrounding tissues. The laser beam can be used continuously (as when cutting) or given in short pulses (as when vaporising an endometrial implant).

Several types of laser are used in medicine. These emit light of different wavelengths and penetrate tissues to different depths. Each type of laser has a different effect due to its wavelength and the amount of energy absorbed by tissues around the lasered area.

The argon laser produces light in the visible green wavelength; this is selectively absorbed by the red pigment in blood (haemoglobin) and is used to coagulate tissues, seal bleeding blood vessels and selectively destroy pigmented lesions.

The carbon dioxide (CO_2) laser is the standard type of laser used to cut tissues. It produces an infrared (invisible) beam which is strongly absorbed by water. This means it can vaporise cells (which are full of water) very easily. By moving a finely focused CO_2 laser beam across tissues, the surgeon can make a neat incision. The laser energy is powerful enough to produce an instant tissue seal so there is no problem with unwanted bleeding. One drawback is that the laser can be passed down only a rigid rod, and may not be able to reach out-of-the-way implants.

The KTP (potassium-titanyl-phosphate) laser produces a beam of emerald green light. Laser energy at this wavelength penetrates more deeply than the CO_2 laser and tissues are easily cut by stroking the fibre tip across the surface. Vaporisation is possible if the tip is held close to endometrial implants, or photo-coagulation (light burns) can be produced by holding the beam slightly farther away. This laser can be passed down flexible tubes and is useful when access to an implant is difficult. Unlike the CO_2 laser, it is not absorbed by water and continues to work in the presence of fluid and blood. Like the argon laser, it is absorbed by blood pigments (haemoglobin, haemosiderin) and it is therefore ideal for treating large chocolate endometriomas that are laden with water and blood pigments. It is also useful when many diffuse, pigmented implants are present.

Laser burns heal quickly with minimal scar tissue formation. Studies using different types of laser have found that:

● The neodymium (nd)-YAG laser is associated with pain relief in 92 per cent of cases, and a 37–47 per cent pregnancy rate when treating small ovarian endometriomas;

● Another type of laser, the argon laser, is associated with a 24–34 per cent pregnancy rate;

● The carbon dioxide laser is associated with a 68 per cent pregnancy rate after surgery;

● The KTP laser is associated with a 37 per cent pregnancy rate after surgery.

For this reason, many operators prefer the carbon dioxide laser for treating mild to moderate endometriosis. It is the most controllable type of laser. The argon laser is more effective at vaporising large endometrial cysts and sealing large blood vessels, while the nd-YAG laser – which can penetrate more deeply into tissues – is sometimes used in the destruction of large endometrial implants.

The use of a laser requires specialist training and careful safety precautions. Laser surgery is employed to:

● divide or vaporise adhesions
● vaporise endometriotic implants
● cut out or drain ovarian endometrial cysts
● improve fertility (reconstructive surgery)
● divide nerves supplying the uterus to relieve pain (see page 100).

What happens during laser treatment? When a laser is used during laparoscopy, two extra abdominal incisions are needed as well as the two standard ones just below the umbilicus and just above the pubic bone. The two extra incisions are made one on either side of the lower abdomen just below the bikini line. These four small cuts are needed for:

- the laparoscope itself (umbilical cut)
- grasping instruments etc for lifting and holding organs (mid-line cut above pubic bone)
- the laser (first lateral cut)
- a venting device that lets smoke and vaporised tissue out of the abdomen and allows irrigating fluid to be added for washing out and cooling the peritoneal cavity (second lateral cut); this incision can also be used for extra cutting instruments.

All incisions will be closed with a single stitch or a staple at the end of the operation (see page 94).

Some surgeons attach the eyepiece of the laparoscope to a video camera so they can watch everything on a screen rather than peering down the laparoscope itself with one eye. This is called video-laparoscopy and gives excellent views of your endometrial lesions.

The laser can also be fitted to the operating channel of the laparoscope so it passes through the same incision. This frees the second lateral incision so that other operating instruments can be inserted.

The use of laser surgery to destroy endometrial lesions is highly effective in relieving symptoms of pelvic pain. The success rate is quoted at 70 per cent. Laser excision of endometrial implants also results in increased chance of subsequent pregnancy (see page 97). For this reason, many surgeons are keen to perform surgical excision of lesions, especially where a patient is suffering from pain or subfertility. Laser surgery seems to give better results than microsurgery (conventional surgery performed under a microscope) for moderate to severe endometriosis.

Laser surgery in peritoneal endometriosis Vaporising an endometrial implant on the abdominal cavity lining with a carbon dioxide laser is very quick.

Initially, any old blood that has collected in the lesion will bubble as it is heated, followed by bubbling of a curdy white material which represents vaporisation of the ectopic endometrial tissue itself. This removes the implant down as far as the underlying level of fatty tissue. As soon as the surgeon sees the fat bubbling, he knows it is time to stop. Water is then added to absorb the CO_2 laser beam for a few seconds and ensure it does not penetrate any deeper. The water also flushes away charred pieces of tissue and clears the surgeon's view.

Laser designs are now so sophisticated that very short laser pulses (ultrapulse mode) can be used like a long knife literally to shave off implants from tricky areas of peritoneum such as those covering the bowel, bladder, ureter or an artery. In these situations, the surgeon will usually take the extra precaution of injecting a volume of salt water behind the lesion. This safety measure separates the lesion from underlying tissues and elevates it on a bleb, or small air bubble (aquadissection) and absorbs the laser beam if it penetrates too deeply (aquaprotection).

In severe cases of peritoneal endometriosis, a course of GnRH agonist before surgery will help to reduce inflammation. However, this usually isn't needed. Unfortunately, lesions can form after laser treatment; these seem to be new lesions at new sites rather than a recurrence of previously removed implants. Hormonal manipulation may help to prevent the return of your endometriosis or may be offered to treat symptoms that recur.

Laser surgery in ovarian endometriosis Superficial ovarian implants are lasered until follicles containing fluid are encountered, or until no further pigmented tissue is seen. Those that are under 2cm across tend to be full of fibrous tissue (fibrotic) and are usually biopsied and then vaporised.

Small fluid-filled ovarian endometriomas that measure 2–3cm across can usually be treated during one procedure, so long as they do not penetrate farther into the ovary than 3cm.

First, a small hole in the top of the cyst measuring 3–4mm across is cut out. Then, the chocolate-coloured fluid is drained off with a suction device and the remaining cavity thoroughly flushed out with water.

Next, the inside wall of the cyst is carefully examined through the laparoscope to ensure that there are no suspicious lesions inside (such as early ovarian tumour) and biopsied. This is essential, as a form of ovarian cancer (endometrioid adenocarcinoma) looks identical to an endometrioma and can be distinguished from it only under a microscope. The wall of the cyst is then vaporised with the laser until no further pigment is seen to minimise the risk of recurrence.

After another thorough washing, the hole this procedure makes in the ovary is left open. There will be no bleeding because the laser beam has cauterised the area.

When cysts measuring more than 3cm across are found, most surgeons prefer to do a two-step procedure (some do this only if the cyst is over 5cm across).

First, the cyst is drained and washed out at laparoscopy as described above for smaller cysts. Then, after an inspection of the inner cyst wall, a biopsy is taken for examination under the microscope.

The cyst is then left in this open, un-lasered state and the woman is given a course of a GnRH agonist for 12 weeks. This usually shrinks the cyst down by at least 50 per cent.

The woman then has a repeat laparoscopy and the residual cyst is examined again. If it has shrunk down to below 3cm, it is lasered as described above. If the cyst is still greater than 3cm across (sometimes 5cm) a different technique is performed to preserve the ovarian anatomy as much as possible.

This different technique involves a partial removal of the part of the cyst that protrudes above the surface of the ovary. This is done by making a circular cut with the laser beam. The inside of the remaining cyst is then re-examined and biopsied.

Next, the inner cyst wall is vaporised with the laser beam, and – instead of being left open – the edges of the cyst are brought together and a special tissue glue is used to seal them together (fibrin sealant). This avoids leaving a large gap that might interfere with the blood supply of the remaining ovarian tissue. The abdominal cavity is then further washed out to remove traces of vaporised tissue (carbon) and glue.

Plain laparoscopic treatment of an endometrioma If you are having only laparoscopy, without laser surgery, your endometrioma will be treated slightly differently. After making a hole and drawing out the fluid contents, the surgeon will inspect the cyst wall. Its capsule will then be stripped from the ovary – rather like peeling an inside-out mushroom – using two pairs of grasping forceps. These strips will then act like the biopsy and be sent for examination under the microscope.

Some surgeons find it easier to remove the cyst wall by first injecting saline behind it. This helps to separate it from underlying tissues (aqua-or hydro-dissection). Any bleeding points in the ovary are sealed using diathermy (coagulation using electricity).

The edges of the remaining hole in the ovary usually meet up, in which case the defect is left to heal. If they don't meet, they may be:

- buzzed with the coagulator so they contract and meet
- glued together with a fibrin sealant
- stapled together with a titanium clip
- or sewn together with a couple of stitches.

Stitching increases the risk of adhesions forming after the operation (see page 98).

Complications Routine laser surgery can be done as an outpatient treatment or on an inpatient basis with up to 48 hours in hospital. If complications occur or if the specialist decides to proceed to an open operation, you will need to stay in longer.

The possible complications of laser surgery are of two types:

- those relating to the laparoscopy
- those relating to the laser treatment.

At the beginning of a laparoscopy, a large-bore needle is introduced into the abdominal cavity, and there is a small risk that this may damage the bowel, bladder or blood vessels. If this happens a laparotomy is then needed to repair the damage. Similarly, the laser beam itself may be inaccurately directed at an endometrial lesion, and cause damage to surrounding structures which then require open repair.

Risks of the operation are increased in women who are very overweight, very underweight or have had previous abdominal surgery (because of scar tissue formation).

There is always, too, a small risk associated with having a general anaesthetic. These risks should be explained to you before the operation by your anaesthetist.

Depending on your circumstances, you may be offered a course of hormonal treatment after your laparoscopy. A six-week course of suppressive therapy to prevent ovulation will help the ovaries to heal where a cyst has been removed.

If you do not wish to try for a pregnancy, you may be prescribed the oral contraceptive pill indefinitely. Alternatively, if you do want a baby you may be encouraged to try right away. There seems to be no difference in pregnancy rates following treatment with laser surgery or treatment with danazol.

Laparoscopy and the carbon dioxide laser have transformed the surgical treatment of endometriosis since the mid-1980s. In skilled hands, virtually any endometrial lesion can be treated, with the woman having minimal disruption to her life.

· *Laparotomy* ·

Conservative Surgery for Endometriosis at Laparotomy is abbreviated to CSEL. This treatment was popular in the 1970s, but the development of laparoscopy means that it is now mainly reserved for:

- severe endometriosis with large endometriomas
- severe endometriosis or adhesions beyond the training or available instruments of a laparoscopic surgeon
- women in whom drug treatment and laparoscopy have failed to improve pelvic pain or subfertility
- cases needing more extensive procedures, such as resection of an invasive bowel nodule
- women who are very overweight, making laparoscopy difficult
- cases in which complications have occurred during laparoscopy.

You will be asked to give the surgeon permission to proceed to CSEL under the same general anaesthetic as that used for your diagnostic or treatment laparoscopy if indicated. Some surgeons prefer to wait three months from the diagnostic laparoscopy so you can have a course of suppressive hormone treatment first.

Laparotomy is as effective as laparoscopy, if not more so. Open operation allows the surgeon a better, direct view of your pelvic organs. This means that small lesions in unusual places are less likely to be overlooked. There is a lower risk of complications such as accidental damage to the bowel, bladder, ureters or Fallopian tubes, and bleeding points are more easily controlled. Because of the larger incision, there is an increased risk of adhesions after the operation.

During CSEL, the surgeon is able to use diathermy or laser surgery, depending on the type of equipment available and his or her expertise. Complete removal of an endometrial implant is just as likely whether the surgeon uses scissors or a laser beam, although many surgeons prefer the laser, as it seals the area to prevent bleeding and guarantees a sterile field. The careful use of diathermy has the same advantages.

What happens during laparotomy

If you need to have a laparotomy for the treatment of your endometriosis, you will have a 10–15cm horizontal incision just below your bikini line. In some women (typically the very overweight, or those who already have a scar in the area) a horizontal incision between your pubic bone and your umbilicus may be necessary.

The surgeon aims to touch your insides as little as possible in order to reduce inflammation and subsequent adhesions (see page 98). Your pelvic cavity will be continually washed out with running saline, too.

The first thing your surgeon may do is to cut a bundle of non-essential nerves in your pelvis (presacral neurectomy). This relieves or decreases pelvic pain in the majority of women (see page 39) but it is not always a routine procedure in this country.

Next, all visible endometrial lesions are removed – using either scissor dissection, diathermy or laser surgery. All adhesions will be cut out and removed where possible, rather than just divided.

Special materials called adhesion barriers are sometimes laid over removed incisions to discourage the formation of adhesions, and the surgeon finally closes the abdominal incision after he is happy that all lesions have been removed, all bleeding has stopped, and the pelvic and abdominal cavities have been thoroughly washed out.

CSEL is successful in alleviating pelvic pain in at least 80 per cent of cases. When endometriosis is linked with infertility, CSEL is followed by an overall pregnancy rate of 52 per cent. This can be broken down according to the stage of disease to pregnancy in:

- 60–75 per cent of women with mild endometriosis
- 50–65 per cent of women with moderate endometriosis
- 39–50 per cent of women with severe endometriosis.

These figures are similar to those for laparoscopy. Thus, the two methods are equally effective in removing endometrial implants.

After your operation, you must ask the surgeon exactly what was found during your laparotomy and what was done, especially if the appendix or an ovary was removed.

Complications of laparotomy

Complications are unusual with CSEL. They are more likely where extensive disease requires surgery to the bowel, bladder, over-large blood vessels, or near the ureters. Possible complications include:

- infection
- excessive blood loss
- accidental damage to bowel, bladder, Fallopian tubes, blood vessels or ureters.

There is also a risk associated with the general anaesthetic.

Endometriosis seems to recur in 15 per cent of women who just have CSEL within three years, and in 35 per cent of women within five years.

Combined medical and surgical treatment

Surgery alone may not be the best treatment for your endometriosis. This may be because:

- non-visible implants are not removed;
- implants over a vital structure (e.g. artery, ureter) may not be totally removed for fear of damage;
- implants may recur or new ones develop;
- adhesions may form afterwards which can reduce fertility.

In several studies involving laparoscopy versus laparoscopy plus danazol, better pregnancy rates were found when using both medical and surgical treatment together (see table on page 98).

Some surgeons, however, feel that this is not the case with laser surgery. Pregnancy rates after laser surgery are as high as 75 per cent (most within eight months), and they feel there is no justification for delaying an attempt at pregnancy by prescribing danazol first.

You must be guided by your own surgeon as to what he or she feels is the right course of action for you.

Pregnancy rates (%) in 6-year trial

Endometriosis	Surgery only	Surgery plus pre-op danazol	% increase with danazol
Mild	73%	85%	+12%
Moderate	56%	69%	+13%
Severe	40%	53%	+13%

From: Rationale for combined medical and surgical treatment of endometriosis. V.C. Buttram in The current status of endometriosis, research and management. Ed I. Brosens and J. Donnez. Parthenon Publishing, 1993.

· *Adhesions and why they form* ·

One of the main drawbacks of abdominal surgery is the risk of adhesions forming after the operation.

Adhesions can be triggered by anything that injures or inflames the peritoneum, including surgery, infection and endometriosis itself.

Damage to the peritoneum is thought to cause release of inflammatory chemicals such as histamine and kinins. These stimulate dilation of nearby blood vessels which start to leak protein-rich fluid from the circulation into surrounding tissues. This fluid is rich in blood-clotting factors, and strands of clotted protein (fibrin) rapidly form in the same way that a graze on your skin quickly seals itself. These thick, clotted strands can stick pelvic organs together. Normally, fibrin is just as quickly broken down by the action of an enzyme, plasmin, so normal healing can occur without adhesion formation.

When endometriosis is present, or when oxygen supplies to the tissues are reduced (such as around a stitch inserted into the ovary) less plasmin is made, so fibrin can build up. In severe cases of injury (major surgery) or inflammation (such as a major infection), so much protein-rich fluid is exuded into the abdomen that the plasmin enzyme cannot keep up with breaking it down. It also seems as if endometriosis triggers the production of higher amounts of fibrin-rich peritoneal fluid to increase the risk of adhesions.

Once the fibrin strands are established, and not dissolved by plasmin, they quickly form a matrix into which blood cells and fibre-producing cells (fibroblasts) become trapped, and tiny blood vessels grow in to produce something similar to a scab or clot.

These fibrous strips mat organs together and eventually contract slightly, like elastic bands, to form what are known as adhesions.

In summary, adhesions are more likely to develop if:

- extensive or repeated surgery is needed

- inflammation is present
- infection occurs
- endometriosis is relatively severe
- tissues receive an inadequate supply of blood and oxygen
- a lot of stitches are needed.

Adhesions form in 55–100 per cent of women after a gynaecological surgical procedure. They can mat pelvic organs together and block the entrance to the Fallopian tubes, reducing the chance of pregnancy. They can also cause pain by tethering organs together. Surgeons try to minimise your risk of developing adhesions by various measures:

- minimising tissue handling
- carefully stopping any bleeding (haemostasis)
- avoiding use of sutures where possible
- using tiny sutures with low tissue irritation
- strictly controlling infection
- using magnification where possible
- keeping tissues moist during the operation
- washing out the abdominal cavity with saline containing a blood clot preventer (heparin) or with tissue enzymes
- using an adhesion barrier – a special material placed over a wound to inhibit adhesions (e.g. Interceed); this is slowly absorbed by the body over a few weeks.

Giving a course of suppressive treatment (e.g. danazol or GnRH agonists) before surgery also seems to reduce adhesion formation in some cases by reducing the amount of active endometriosis and inflammation present at the time of operation.

Drug treatment on its own will not touch adhesions once they have formed. The only way to remove them is to cut them out or to vaporise them with a laser.

· *Surgery to relieve pain* ·

Removing endometrial lesions and adhesions and emptying ovarian endometriomas can help to relieve pain for up to one year in as many as 75 per cent of patients. Where this has not helped, interrupting the nerve pathways that transmit pain sensations can provide relief from severely painful periods and intractable pelvic pain in many sufferers.

Pelvic pain sensations are mainly passed through a plexus called the presacral nerve, which lies over the fourth and fifth lumbar vertebrae. This can be cut using traditional surgical or modern laser techniques, such as presacral neurectomy.

In 11 patients treated with both conservative surgery and presacral neurectomy, 45 per cent had excellent pain relief and 91 per cent showed improvement. This can compared with a group of 64 women who had surgery alone, in which 28 per cent had excellent pain relief and 75 per cent showed improvement.

Laser uterine nerve ablation (LUNA) is a similar technique in which the nerve fibres are buzzed and sealed with a laser. LUNA has a 60–80 per cent success rate in relieving severe dysmenorrhoea and constant pelvic pain.

The presacral nerve often has several trunks, so the surgeon needs to make sure they are all identified. Sometimes nerve fibres are missed and pain continues, although it is usually diminished.

An alternative is to cut the nerves at the junction of the uterus and uterosacral ligaments. This is called uterosacral neurectomy.

· *After an operation* ·

The first thing you need to do when you have recovered from the operation is to ask your surgeon exactly what was found and what was done:

- Were your ovaries and Fallopian tubes healthy?
- Did you have an ovarian endometrioma – if so, how big?
- Did you have many adhesions?
- Was your bowel or bladder involved in the disease?
- What stage is your endometriosis?
- What are the results of any biopsies?
- Were any nerves cut to relieve your pain?
- Was your appendix removed routinely?
- What further treatment is recommended?

To this list add any other questions you may have.

· *Radical surgery* ·

Radical surgery – involving removal of organs such as the womb and/or ovaries and Fallopian tubes – is sometimes the best course of action if a woman's family is complete, and if other less drastic measures have failed.

Surgical castration – removal of the ovaries – was formerly one of the most effective treatments for endometriosis as the implants are oestrogen-dependent. A reversible form of medical castration is now available: GnRH agonists (see page 79). However, this treatment is recommended only for a six-month course at present due to the thinning effects on bone. The introduction of combined drug treatments (added-back oestrogen, progestogen or danazol) may change the time constraints in future.

Radical surgery is covered in Chapter 20.

15

INFERTILITY

Infertility is one of the most controversial and frustrating problems associated with endometriosis. It is commonly stated that between 25 and 50 per cent of infertile women have endometriosis and that 30–50 per cent of women with endometriosis are infertile.

However, these figures are based on studies done in the 1930s and 1940s, on women who had endometriosis diagnosed at laparotomy. When their notes were reviewed by later researchers, it was discovered that 30 per cent of these women had never had children, some women were unable to have as many children as they would wish, and some had suffered from miscarriages. This is how the widely accepted statement that '30–50 per cent of women with endometriosis are infertile' originated. The good news is that it is likely to be an overestimate for several reasons:

● The studies were done before laparoscopy was available; they are based on women whose symptoms were severe enough to warrant laparotomy. Women with milder symptoms were not included.
● The studies were done at a time when minimal and mild endometriosis were underestimated, and atypical lesions were unrecognised. The women with milder disease were not considered to have the disease.
● The diagnoses of endometriosis and infertility were not made in the same women at the same time; one condition simply could have followed the other rather than being causally connected.

In fact, researchers still don't know the true incidence of endometriosis within the female population, the frequency of infertility within the general population, or how often endometriosis and infertility are linked. Until this link is identified, the question of which causes which is also in dispute.

In 20–50 per cent of couples investigated for infertility the female partner is found to have endometriosis. By comparison, the generally accepted incidence of endometriosis in women of reproductive age is only 10 per cent (although this figure may well be an underestimate – see page 2). This difference has led many researchers to assume that the presence of ectopic endometrial implants is in some way responsible for the difficulty in conceiving. Others argue that whereas this observation suggests an association between endometriosis and infertility, it does not show that endometriosis causes it.

Many studies suggest that women with endometriosis spontaneously conceive at the same rate as infertile women without endometriosis.

It is important to remember that most women with endometriosis are not sterile; they just take longer to get pregnant, with more treatment cycles needed if undergoing fertility treatment. 'Subfertility' is therefore a more accurate description of their condition than the totally negative term 'infertility'.

Another important factor is that many subfertile women with endometriosis are in their mid-to late-30s – both because it is now more common to delay parenthood and because this is the decade when endometriosis is most commonly diagnosed. Significant numbers are therefore thought to have problems conceiving as a result of the natural age-related decline in fertility rather than as a result of endometriosis itself:

Age of woman	Average time to pregnancy	Monthly chance of pregnancy with artificial insemination
25 years	2–3 months	11%
35 years	6 months or longer	6.5%

Doctors have tried to link severity of endometriosis with the subsequent chance of pregnancy, but this approach is difficult. The staging system used to classify endometriosis (revised American Fertility Society – see page 62) is itself based on clinical findings that are thought to increase the risk of infertility. Despite this, there is no proven link between subfertility and the amount of endometriosis present.

Some researchers feel that the AFS classification system falls down by mixing factors such as number and size of peritoneal implants, with mechanical factors such as presence of adhesions and endometriomas. This makes it more difficult to compare the severity of endometriosis with future chance of pregnancy. For this reason, some doctors prefer to consider two types of infertility associated with endometriosis:

• infertility in women who have only endometrial implants
• infertility in women with distortion of their reproductive organs through ovarian endometriomas, Fallopian tube obstruction or adhesions.

Many women with no obvious adhesions or distortion of the reproductive organs – classified as having only mild or minimal endometriosis – are still subfertile, however. This is what makes researching the link between subfertility and endometriosis so frustrating.

Theories linking subfertility with endometriosis

Many theories have been suggested to explain why endometriosis is statistically linked with subfertility. The possible mechanisms include:

- anatomical distortion and tubal obstruction
- Fallopian tube dysfunction
- failure of egg capture after ovulation
- ovarian dysfunction
- luteinised unruptured follicle (LUF) syndrome (see page 105)
- high levels of prolactin hormone
- recurrent, unrecognised, spontaneous miscarriage at an early stage of embryo development
- altered immunity
- hostility to egg of inflammatory chemicals in intraperitoneal fluid
- abnormal hormone levels before and after ovulation
- abnormal interaction between sperm and egg which prevents fertilisation
- abnormal interaction between fertilised egg and normal endometrium which prevents implantation
- defective luteal phase of the menstrual cycle.

None of these theories are backed by sufficient data to prove a link with endometriosis and subfertility and more than one mechanism may be involved. It is possible that there is no link whatever – merely a chance association. The most popular theories are reviewed below.

Anatomical distortion

This is one of the earliest theories linking subfertility and endometriosis. Ovaries can be distorted by large chocolate-coloured cysts, the finger-like ends (fimbriae) of the Fallopian tubes can be damaged by active lesions to form club-like remnants, and the end of the tube can be blocked by adhesions. In rare cases, the inner bore of the Fallopian tubes can be blocked as well. Reconstructive surgery to restore a semblance of normal anatomy seems to increase the chance of pregnancy by at least 30 per cent.

Fallopian tube dysfunction

The fluid inside the Fallopian tubes is continuous with that in the peritoneal cavity.

There is a theory that hormone-like inflammatory chemicals (prostaglandins) secreted by ectopic endometrial tissue may enter the

Fallopian tubes and alter transport of the sperm or egg to reduce the chance of conception. Certainly there are higher levels of prostaglandins in the peritoneal fluid of women with endometriosis. Egg and sperm transport in the Fallopian tubes, however, are due mainly to the action of cilia, and no evidence has yet been found that this action is affected by prostaglandins. Moreover, drugs that inhibit prostaglandin production do not have an obvious effect on fertility.

Failure of egg capture

One research group found that an unidentified substance in the peritoneal fluid of women with endometriosis reduced fertility in hamsters. It triggered formation of a smooth membrane over the cilia in the hamsters' Fallopian tubes. This unidentified factor prevented a newly ovulated egg from attaching to the Fallopian tube and was dubbed the ovum capture inhibitor (OCI). When the membrane was gently removed from the cilia, normal ovum capture resumed. This experiment has not been duplicated by other researchers, and it is not known if a similar membrane forms in humans.

Ovarian dysfunction

Some researchers believe there are subtle ovulatory defects in subfertile women with endometriosis, though they are unable to say exactly what these are. Their theory is based on the observation that endometriosis is more common in women who have had a long series of ovulatory cycles without pregnancy. This situation also increases the incidence of retrograde menstruation, however (see page 18) – a likely cause of endometriosis itself.

Some women with endometriosis do not ovulate in some cycles. A follicle fails to develop properly, ovulation fails and the luteal cyst does not form. But although some women with endometriosis are found to have these anovulatory cycles, so do women without endometriosis. It is estimated that, on average, 1 in 13 cycles is normally anovulatory. The only evidence a woman may have of the event is a slightly heavier period which comes on slightly earlier (see page 11). There is no evidence that lack of ovulation is the main cause of endometriosis-associated subfertility.

A few researchers have found lower levels of progesterone in the second half of the menstrual cycle in infertile women with endometriosis (luteal phase defects) but other researchers dispute this. Also, treatment with fertility drugs that overcome luteal phase deficiency (e.g. clomiphene, progesterone suppositories) do not seem to increase the success rate for each cycle of treatment.

Most doctors believe that the luteal phase of the menstrual cycle is normal in most women with endometriosis, based on comparisons between development of normal endometrium and the mid-cycle surge of leutinising hormone (LH) from the pituitary gland (see page 7).

LUF syndrome

After an egg is released, its follicle usually collapses and fills with blood. It is then infiltrated with cells that start to produce the hormone progesterone. The ruptured follicle is then converted into the corpus luteum (see page 9).

Some researchers believe that a ripe egg can fail to discharge and remain trapped inside its follicle. The follicle is then thought to undergo its usual leutinised changes to form the corpus luteum, and still produces progesterone, but remains unruptured. This theory is attractive, for if this does occur, standard fertility tests would fail to pick it up. Normal cyclical changes in cervical mucus, body temperature, endometrial tissues and blood hormone levels would still suggest that ovulation had occurred. It would therefore neatly explain the reduced fertility with normal base-line tests that can occur in endometriosis.

Some studies suggest that laparoscopic findings suggestive of LUF syndrome are more common in women with endometriosis than those without; other studies show no statistically significant differences.

Year	*% of women with evidence of LUF syndrome at laparoscopy*	
	women with endometriosis	*women without endometriosis*
1978	79	6
1980		
	57 – 67%	
	59 – 64%	
1980	43 – 77%	52 – 58%
1982	28%	9%
1983	16 – 61%	10 – 28%
1984	62 – 72%	21 – 72%

High prolactin levels

Prolactin is another hormone produced by the pituitary gland. It is released in highest quantities during the end of pregnancy, when it is responsible for stimulating and maintaining breast milk production.

Sometimes, an overgrowth of the pituitary gland can cause high levels of prolactin hormone outside of pregnancy. Symptoms include lack of sex drive, secretion of a milky discharge from the nipples, lack of periods (amenorrhoea) – and lowered fertility.

Because raised levels of prolactin (prolactinaemia) are linked with subfertility, several researchers have measured prolactin levels in women with endometriosis:

Year	Number of women with endometriosis	% with raised prolactin	% with milky breast discharge
1978	9	11%	55%
1980	14	21%	0%
1982	14	21%	–
1984	55	36%	–

These studies would suggest that at least some women with endometriosis may have subfertility due to raised prolactin levels.

Studies comparing average prolactin levels in women with and without endometriosis show no significant differences, however.

Prolactin hormone levels are usually measured routinely in women with subfertility (except when they are ovulating). If your level is found to be high, your doctor may suggest treatment with a drug (bromocriptine) that acts on the pituitary gland to lower prolactin secretion.

It is worth asking your doctor what your prolactin level is. Sometimes the hormone is measured by an especially alert GP; sometimes it is requested by the hospital. If both sides think the other has done it, it is easily forgotten – it's best to check.

Recurrent miscarriage

Overall, it is estimated that between 20 and 80 per cent of newly fertilised eggs fail to implant in the uterine wall. This is known as pre-implantation wastage and occurs before conception is medically or legally recognised. Of those fertilised eggs that do successfully implant and start to produce a placenta, around 30 per cent miscarry – most before the mother is aware that she is pregnant. The only sign may be that the next period is slightly later or heavier than usual.

Some researchers have suggested that a subfertile woman is more likely to have a higher rate of spontaneous miscarriages after treatment for endometriosis than before her diagnosis for the disease. This may be because they are more alert to signs of pregnancy, and may recognise their pregnancy earlier than before. Also, the rate of spontaneous miscarriage increases with age and these patients are obviously older than when they were pregnant before.

Endometriosis is also more common in women aged 30–40, a factor that complicates this theory even further.

Recent studies have found a similar risk of spontaneous miscarriage in subfertile women both with and without endometriosis. Highly sensitive pregnancy tests have also failed to diagnose early spontaneous miscarriage in subfertile women with endometriosis, which seems to knock this theory soundly on the head.

Altered immunity

Many abnormalities of the immune system have been described in women with endometriosis (see page 26). None of these are consistent, however, and none seems to increase the risk of subfertility.

Some researchers have found that women with endometriosis have self-antibodies directed against their endometrial glands. These may play a role in preventing implantation of a fertilised egg, but again their presence is not consistent.

The immune system is currently undergoing intense research activity. If altered immune function could be linked with subfertility, it is likely that scientists will come up with a treatment to combat it.

Peritoneal fluid inflammation

The peritoneal fluid contains scavenger white cells (leukocytes, macrophages) with several functions:

- removal of bacteria that find their way up the female genital tract
- removal of sperm swimming out of the Fallopian tubes
- mopping up the products of retrograde menstruation.

Infertile women with endometriosis seem to have a higher number of scavenger white cells in their peritoneal fluid than fertile women. In particular, they seem to have more activated macrophages (see page 22) which are stimulated by the presence of retrograde menstruation.

These scavenger cells are likely to enter a Fallopian tube and attack sperm, killing them or slowing them down before they can reach the egg. Activated macrophages may also attack a newly released egg and affect its transportation down the Fallopian tube. If fertilisation does occur, they may somehow prevent implantation into the endometrium or interfere with early embryo/placenta development.

These theories all have some data to support them, but are by no means widely accepted. Infertile women with endometriosis also have evidence of increased low-key, sterile, inflammatory secretions in their peritoneal fluid. When compared with fertile women without endometriosis, they have an increased volume of peritoneal fluid which contains higher concentrations of scavenger cell enzymes, inflammatory chemicals and cell simulating growth factors.

These inflammatory chemicals are likely to be hostile to a freshly released egg. They may interfere with fertilisation by breaking down sperm-attracting chemicals released by the egg or by changing its outer shell. Research is currently directed at this area of investigation.

You still have a good chance of pregnancy

Couples in which the female partner has endometriosis are not infertile. They are subfertile. This means you have a lower monthly chance of conception, so you have to try for longer before conception occurs. Subfertility is usually diagnosed when you have failed to conceive after twelve months of regular, unprotected intercourse.

Your best friend is time. Out of every 100 women with endometriosis who try to conceive without any treatment whatsoever, between one and three will successfully become pregnant per month. This compares with an average 20 per cent chance of pregnancy per month in couples who have normal fertility.

Doctors now assess how successful fertility treatments are by calculating their monthly fecundity rate. This is worked out by calculating the total number of pregnancies achieved and dividing it by the number of months of pregnancy exposure (can be multiplied by 100 to give a percentage). All couples treated with a fertility technique are included in the calculation – even those who are lost to follow-up; these are included as if they failed to conceive.

Various trials show the following encouraging annual pregnancy rates (and related monthly fecundity) for women with mild endometriosis, who receive no treatment but time (so-called expectant treatment!):

Number of women in study	Overall % who successfully conceived	monthly fecundity (chance of conception per month)
17	64.7%	0.050 (5%)
18	72.2%	0.102 (10.2%)
28	50%	0.111 (11.1%)
31	61.2%	0.083 (8.3%)
34	52.9%	0.057 (5.7%)

These pregnancy rates were recorded over differing periods of time, but for the total 128 women, it is estimated that 50.3 per cent became pregnant within one year. In couples of normal fertility, most (i.e. almost 100 per cent) would expect to conceive within one year.

· *Subfertility statistics* ·

If you are suffering from subfertility, it is important to remember that you are not alone. Subfertility is the commonest reason for referral to hospital in people under the age of 40. One in 20 males (5 per cent) is subfertile at any one time and 25 per cent of women will experience some form of reduced fertility – one in eight while trying for their first baby. Only 3 per cent of women are involuntarily childless, but 6 per cent are unable to have as many children as they would wish.

Male factors are significant in around 20 per cent of couples who are subfertile. Female ovulatory failure (anovulation) accounts for 25 per cent of cases, Fallopian tubal damage (such as blockage) for around 10 per cent and endometriosis for between 20 and 50 per cent of cases. These figures do not add up to 100 per cent because sometimes more than one factor is involved.

Causes of subfertility remain unexplained in a significant number of cases despite extensive investigation. New research suggests that antibodies against sperm, or faulty sperm enzymes needed for fertilisation (acrosome reaction) may be involved.

· *Fertilisation* ·

Your window of fertility in each cycle is very short. An egg is fresh enough for fertilisation during only the first 48 hours after ovulation. In a regular 28-day cycle, this will centre around day 14, where day 1 is counted as the first day of menstrual bleeding. To maximise your chances of conception, you should aim to make love during the seven-day fertile phase of your menstrual cycle. This is the five days before ovulation is expected, and the two days just after ovulation. The egg can be fertilised only during the 48 hours immediately after ovulation. Because sperm can remain potent inside you for about five days and the egg is fresh enough for fertilization for two days, any sperm that arrives more than five days before ovulation or more than two days after it is unlikely to cause conception.

Sadly, a national survey found that 57 per cent of women and 76 per cent of men did not know that a woman is most fertile in the middle of her menstrual cycle.

An ovulation prediction kit will help you to time your fertile phase most accurately.

· *Tests for subfertility* ·

Examination of a subfertile couple may reveal anatomical abnormalities such as malformed pelvic organs or, in the male, scrotal varicose veins (varicocoeles) which overheat the testes and affect sperm production. Some anatomical problems can be corrected surgically; for example, varicocoeles can be cut out or sealed with sclerosing injections. Your own doctor will advise you on any unusual findings and suggested treatment options.

The simplest fertility test is for a woman to take her temperature every morning before getting out of bed.

Central body temperature goes up by a fraction of a degree when ovulation occurs; this is a progesterone effect. A special fertility (ultra-sensitive) thermometer is needed and the temperature must be taken immediately on waking every morning, before getting out of bed. Some doctors question the value of temperature charts and the stress they may place on subfertile women. An ovulation predictor kit (which measures hormones in urine) may be better.

Several blood tests are needed to assess your various reproductive hormone levels. These are best done on day 21 of your cycle (when blood progesterone levels will be highest if you have ovulated). At the same time, your partner may be asked to provide a semen sample for analysis. This sample needs to be fresh and the laboratory must be on stand-by to receive it and analyse it immediately before sperm start to become sluggish or die.

If low sperm count and abnormal hormone levels are ruled out, the next step is often a post-coital test. This involves seeing a doctor the morning after a sexually active 'night before' – usually just before you are expected to ovulate, when your cervical mucus is sperm-friendly. The doctor will remove a sample of mucus from your cervix (painless, just like having a cervical smear) and examine it under the microscope. If active, live sperm are seen, the test is normal.

If no sperm are seen, or if large numbers of abnormal or sluggish sperm are encountered, there may be a problem such as:

- an abnormality with your partner's sperm
- your love-making technique
- an incompatibility between you and your partner's sperm such as anti-sperm antibodies.

These findings will need professional follow-up.

If you have a post-coital test and it is normal, you may be booked straight in for a diagnostic laparoscopy. Sometimes this may be preceded by a few more tests, such as an ultrasound scan (see page 121), a dye-X-ray test to flush the Fallopian tubes through and establish that they are unobstructed (hysterosalpingogram) or a new technique, falloposcopy. This involves inserting a flexible telescope into the Fallopian tubes via the uterus – usually when a previous diagnosis of Fallopian tube disease has been made. Doctors can then assess the extent of internal scarring (from previous pelvic inflammatory disease, surgery or endometriosis) and determine whether tubal surgery would help. Falloposcopy can also be used to clear the uterine end of the tubes of up to 40 per cent obstruction due to debris.

Occasionally, the hypothalamo-pituitary-gonadal axis (see page 79) is assessed to make sure your hypothalamus and pituitary gland are kick-starting your ovaries properly.

GnRH is secreted in pulses every one to four hours from the hypothalamus in the brain, then passes down to stimulate the pituitary gland just beneath it (see page 79).

The pituitary responds by releasing pulses of follicle stimulating hormone (FSH) and luteinising hormone (LH) which stimulate egg development in the ovaries. This hormone system can be checked for responsiveness by giving you an injection of GnRH and measuring the blood levels of the other hormones over the following hour.

Other tests may be done on your partner's sperm to see if they can fertilise an egg properly in a test-tube. Some sperm lack the enzymes needed for this, or fail to release them at the right time. These specialist tests are available in only a few centres.

Treatment of subfertility associated with endometriosis

Your treatment for subfertility will very much depend upon the stage of your disease – whether it is minimal, mild, moderate or severe.

If your endometriosis is moderate or severe, with mechanical distortion of your reproductive organs (such as ovarian endometrioma, blocked Fallopian tubes, adhesions), most gynaecologists would recommend reconstructive surgery in an attempt to restore your anatomy to normal. This can be done with a traditional laparotomy or newer endoscopic techniques – with or without laser vaporisation.

If endometrial implants are present only on your peritoneal membrane (diagnosed through laparoscopy) the options are much wider. Depending on severity, medical treatment can include:

- danazol
- gestrinone
- progestogens
- GnRH agonist
- conservative surgery with diathermy
- laser vaporisation
- assisted fertility techniques.

· *Treatment successes* ·

The medical treatment of subfertility has widely differing success rates of between 10 and 65 per cent.

Trials consistently suggest that women with minimal or mild endometriosis are no more likely to get pregnant if they receive treatment than if they continue trying for a pregnancy on a wait-and-see basis. This second approach is just as likely to have a successful outcome as taking a course of danazol, gestrinone, medroxyprogesterone acetate or GnRH agonist first. If your only problem is subfertility, non-interference is perhaps the best option. If you are in pain, however, drug treatment will significantly improve your symptoms without seeming to affect your fertility in the long run.

In a study involving women with minimal endometriosis, one random group was given danazol, while the other half were given no treatment. The pregnancy rates were 36 per cent in the treated group and 57 per cent in the non-treated group. Other trials involving danazol, MPA and wait-and-see groups also show little difference to chose between them. In fact some results suggest that women who are on no treatment may become pregnant sooner (within ten months) than those receiving treatment (17–18 months). This can be disheartening for researchers and couples alike.

Progestogen treatment for subfertility

In women with mild endometriosis, studies have failed to show a consistent beneficial increase in pregnancy rates after treatment with progestogens. This finding is common to all other drugs (e.g. danazol, gestrinone, GnRH agonists) used in the treatment of endometriosis-associated subfertility.

In one of the most hopeful early studies (1976), 12 out of 26 women with endometriosis-associated subfertility became pregnant after a three-month course of medroxyprogesterone acetate. The researchers claimed that 90 per cent of women whose husbands were fertile successfully conceived during this trial.

A similar trial involving nine months' treatment with dydrogesterone resulted in 10 out of 19 women (53 per cent) becoming pregnant afterwards (although, sadly, two women had a miscarriage).

Danazol treatment for subfertility

In women with mild endometriosis, studies have failed to show an increase in pregnancy rates after treatment with danazol. These findings are common to all other drugs used in the treatment of endometriosis-associated subfertility.

Where treatment with danazol is tried, most spontaneous conceptions occur soon after the drug is stopped. In one early study (1978), which reported an overall 72 per cent pregnancy rate within three years, most conceptions (59 per cent) occurred within the first six months after stopping the drug, and a total of 77 per cent occurred within one year.

Gestrinone treatment for subfertility

In a trial involving 37 women (1987) with minimal or mild endometriosis, 20 were given active gestrinone, and 17 received inactive pretend treatment (a placebo). After one year, results were virtually identical, with successful pregnancy in 25 per cent of women receiving gestrinone and 24 per cent of women on placebo. Another placebo-controlled trial in women with non-symptomatic endometriosis found a pregnancy rate of 25 per cent in women receiving gestrinone, compared with 30 per cent in women on the placebo.

Similar studies involving women with unexplained subfertility show that the likelihood of pregnancy with or without treatment seems to be the same whether or not endometriosis is present.

One trial gave 20 women with proven endometriosis a dose of 5mg gestrinone twice weekly for four – eight months. By the third month, symptoms had disappeared in all patients and, of nine women who wanted a baby, five were pregnant within one year.

Gestrinone is excellent at relieving symptoms of pain. Like other drug treatments, however, it has yet to prove itself in overcoming subfertility in women with mild endometriosis.

Most importantly, pregnancy can occur as soon as treatment with gestrinone is stopped. In one trial, 15 per cent of women conceived during their first month after treatment finished.

GnRH treatment for subfertility

A large trial (1992) has shown that, for women with minimal or mild endometriosis, treatment with a GnRH agonist is no more likely to help conception than a wait-and-see approach: 30 per cent of women receiving GnRH agonists, compared with 36 per cent of women given no treatment. More importantly, 10 women in the no-treatment group became pregnant within the first six months after their diagnostic laparoscopy – the time when their colleagues on GnRH agonists had ovulation suppressed (and were using contraception during treatment). Perhaps this was time wasted?

The story is slightly different for women with moderate to severe endometriosis. Treatment with a GnRH agonist for six months before an assisted conception technique (see page 79) was found to increase significantly the number of healthy eggs retrieved. Pregnancy rates per *in vitro* fertilisation treatment cycle were 30 per cent for women with moderate disease and 35 per cent for women with severe disease.

In another trial in which one group of women received a six-month course of a GnRH agonist before assisted conception techniques, 33 per cent became pregnant per treatment cycle compared with only 5 per cent of women who did not receive any drugs first. This is true only for moderate to severe disease, however: women with minimal to mild disease seem to show no benefit from GnRH treatment first.

Laparotomy treatment for subfertility

When endometriosis is linked with infertility, conservative surgery at laparotomy (see page 95) is followed by pregnancy in:

- 75 per cent of women with mild endometriosis
- 65 per cent of women with moderate endometriosis
- 50 per cent of women with severe endometriosis.

These figures are similar to those for laparoscopy, and it is thought to be the removal of endometrial implants that is important, rather than the technique used.

There is no difference in pregnancy rates following treatment with laser surgery or treatment with danazol. This means there is no justification for delaying pregnancy with suppressive danazol treatment after laser therapy in a woman suffering from infertility.

Treatment	Year	Extent of endometriosis	Number of women	Number pregnant	%
None	1982	mild	18	13	72%
	1982	mild	28	14	50%
	1983	mild	31	19	61%
	1985	mild	34	18	53%
Danazol	1982	mild	20	6	30%
	1982	mild	12	4	33%
GnRH agonist	1992	mild	35	17	61%
Conservative surgery	1979	mild	88	61	69%
	1981	mild	45	28	62%
	1982	mild	42	32	76%
	1983	mild	44	26	52%
	1984	mild	20	8	40%
Laser vaporisation	1987	mild	45	18	40%
	1989	mild	39	28	72%

Unfortunately, no therapy specifically directed towards removing ectopic endometrial implants has been shown significantly to improve the chance of conception for a couple with endometriosis-associated subfertility. Researchers argue that when the monthly fecundity (number of pregnancies divided by number of months of pregnancy exposure) is calculated, there is no apparent advantage of any particular medical or surgical treatment – at least in the milder forms of endometriosis.

The combination of medical and surgical treatments does not seem to improve the chance of success. This approach must also balance the use of a drug to suppress ovulation against the amount of time lost before conception is tried for. Time is always your best friend. This is why many doctors are now leaning towards assisted conception techniques, especially in older women.

· *New approaches* ·

Sadly, no properly controlled studies to date have shown that drug treatment is likely to improve the chance of conception in endometriosis-associated subfertility. Some experts have suggested using the following treatment regime in young women with mild endometriosis, who are subfertile but not suffering unduly with pain:

- diagnostic laparoscopy
- 6–12 months' 'wait-and-see' with no treatment, during which 20 per cent of women are likely to conceive
- repeat laparoscopy with surgery and/or drugs if disease has progressed
- further wait-and-see time
- assisted conception techniques.

· *Assisted conception techniques* ·

The subfertility that can occur in women with endometriosis is essentially unexplained. There are no definitive mechanisms to explain its cause and no definitive treatments guaranteed to overcome it.

In view of this, specialists are starting to ignore the fact that a woman has endometriosis and offer treatment as if the disease were not present. Attempts are made to increase fertility in non-specific ways. Some of the techniques used have been given exotic sounding names:

- controlled ovarian over-stimulation (fertility drugs)
- intra-uterine insemination
- SUZI – SubZonal Insemination (injection of a single sperm into an egg in a test-tube)

- TUFT – Trans-Uterine Fallopian Transfer of a test-tube fertilised egg
- GIFT – Gamete Intra-Fallopian Transfer – in which gametes (sperm and eggs) are flushed into the Fallopian tubes
- TET – Tubal Embryo Transfer of a fertilised egg
- PROST – ProNuclear Stage Tubal Transfer
- ZIFT – Zygote Intra-Fallopian Tube Transfer of a developing embryo
- DIPI – Direct Intra-Peritoneal Insemination of sperm
- POST – Peritoneal Oocyte and Sperm Transfer.

Most studies suggest that women with minimal or mild endometriosis have a similar pregnancy success rate following assisted conception techniques as women without the disease. This is especially true when egg retrieval techniques are used (e.g. harvested via laparoscope; ultrasound guided egg pick-up).

Only one trial so far has suggested otherwise. A group of 91 women underwent artificial insemination with donor sperm because of their partners' infertility (absent or extremely low sperm count). Out of 84 women without endometriosis, 46 pregnancies occurred in a total of 380 exposures, giving a monthly fecundity of 12 per cent. Among the seven women with minimal endometriosis, two pregnancies occurred (in the same patient) out of a total of 56 exposures, giving a monthly fecundity of 3.6 per cent. As the number of women with endometriosis in this study is low, this result could be due to chance. In another study involving ten women with mild endometriosis undergoing artificial insemination, nine achieved pregnancy.

Pregnancy rates are unfortunately lower in women with moderate to severe endometriosis who undergo assisted conception techniques. There may also be an increased risk of spontaneous early miscarriage when endometriosis is advanced. One study found a miscarriage rate of 15 per cent in the normal population, raised to an average of 36 per cent in women with endometriosis. The reasons are still unknown but may include:

- an as-yet undetected problem with the egg, peritoneal fluid or developing embryo
- immune system malfunctions
- defect in normal womb lining, preventing implantation of the fertilised egg or blocking its development.

The success rates of *in vitro* (test tube) fertilisation/embryo transfer (IVF/ET) techniques in mild endometriosis depend on the age of the woman and the experience of the clinic.

In a woman of 28 years, the pregnancy rate per treatment cycle is around 22 per cent, at 32 years it's 15 per cent and at 40 it falls to 9.5 per cent. Miscarriage rates increase with age, so the take-home-baby rate is less. Overall, few clinics achieve clinical pregnancy rates higher than 20 per cent.

If you are referred to a specialist clinic, it is important to find out what their quoted success rate is.

Fertility drugs stimulate natural hormone production to trigger ovulation but they also entail the risk release of more than one egg (super-ovulation) and multiple births are well-known risks. The drug clomiphene is used in women who fail to ovulate. It stimulates follicle ripening in 75 per cent of eligible women, and 35 per cent of these will become pregnant. The risk of twins, however, is 5 per cent (normal incidence is $1\frac{1}{4}$ per cent).

Another technique uses hormones extracted from the urine of menopausal women. This provides natural follicle-stimulating hormone (FSH) to trigger follicular development and leutinising hormone (LH) to encourage ripening and release of an egg. In women who are eligible for this treatment, 75–90 per cent will ovulate and 35 per cent will achieve pregnancy. However, the risk of multiple pregnancy is 35 per cent. A newer technique is the delivery of GnRH in pulses (to mimic its natural release) directly into a woman's subcutaneous fat via a pump and fine needle. This triggers ovulation in 90 per cent of menstrual cycles and after six months 90 per cent of patients are pregnant.

Many other treatment advances have been made. GIFT (Gamete Intra-Fallopian Transfer – in which sperm and eggs are flushed into the Fallopian tubes) has a success rate of 21–25 per cent per treatment cycle (multiple pregnancy rate 21 per cent). As a bonus, any endometriomas present in the ovary can be aspirated at the same time as the egg is laparoscopically retrieved from its ripe follicle.

DIPI (Direct Intra-Peritoneal Insemination) has a success rate of 10 per cent per treatment cycle, and POST (Peritoneal Oocyte and Sperm Transfer) is successful in 25 per cent of treatment cycles. The following state-of-the-art techniques have success rates varying from 17 to 37 per cent – again, in women without endometriosis. These include SUZI, TUFT, TET, PROST and ZIFT (see page 116).

These assisted conception techniques have advantages over the expectant approach of waiting for a spontaneous pregnancy. They do one or more of the following:

- bypass one or more of the possible mechanisms that are linked with subfertility in endometriosis
- increase the chance of ovulation, and therefore of conception
- overcome any distortion of the reproductive organs (e.g. endometrioma, blocked Fallopian tubes) if eggs are retrieved, fertilised in the laboratory and subsequently replaced in the reproductive tract
- increase the number of fertile sperm exposed to the egg and guarantee sperm-egg interactions
- result in higher levels of reproductive hormones.

Controlled ovarian overstimulation (to kick-start ovulation) plus deposition of fresh sperm straight into the uterus is the most widely practised technique. It is relatively cheap and less invasive than other techniques. It also saves on time for older women whose natural fertility is declining.

· *Don't rush into pregnancy* ·

Because decreased fertility can result as endometriosis progresses, and because the disease tends to worsen over time, some doctors feel it is important that treatment be started soon after diagnosis to improve your chances of a future pregnancy. Others feel that treatment only damps down the disease in the short term, and as all drugs carry some risks, women with mild disease should follow a wait-and-see approach. In general, women with endometriosis should not postpone motherhood unduly if they wish to have a family. Postponement could reduce your future chances of success. Having said that, it is important not to rush headlong into starting a family if it is not right for you – or if you are not ready yet. Many counsellors recommend the use of oral contraceptive pills (or danazol) to buy you time while you decide whether or not you want to have a child – and if so, when.

· *Self help* ·

The following simple tips may help to improve fertility:

● The scrotum needs to be 4°C cooler than body temperature. Males should wear cotton boxer shorts and loose-fitting trousers. Daily cold water douching of the testicles is recommended by some experts.
● Both partners should stop smoking. Smokers are twice as likely to be subfertile as non-smokers.
● Cut out alcohol. 40 per cent of male infertility has been linked to only a moderate alcohol intake. Evidence points to a similar alcohol association in women; it seems to hasten degeneration of eggs in the ovary.
● Decrease your consumption of caffeine. A study has shown an impressive link between subfertility and drinking more than eight cups of coffee per day. Drinking around three cups of caffeine-containing drinks per day is probably harmless.
● Men should supplement their diet with a multinutrient vitamin containing zinc and vitamins E, C, betacarotene and B12.
● Women should supplement their diet with a multinutrient supplement containing folic acid and vitamin B12.
● Improve your general fitness and in particular ensure that your weight is in the normal range.
● Learn to beat stress with relaxation techniques and try, for example, aromatherapy, homeopathy, acupuncture.

16

ECTOPIC PREGNANCY

An ectopic pregnancy is one that develops outside its normal site. It occurs when a fertilised egg gets stuck during its descent into the womb. The most common place for an ectopic pregnancy to implant is inside a Fallopian tube, usually in the inner one-third where the bore is most narrow. Fertilised eggs have been known to develop in the ovary or inside the abdominal cavity, however, and rarely, in the cervix.

Because endometriosis can damage the Fallopian tubes, or partially block them, affected women can develop an ectopic pregnancy.

· *How common is ectopic pregnancy?* ·

One in every 200 recognised pregnancies in the general population is ectopic. It seems to be increasing in frequency, with the incidence in some parts of the UK found to be as high as one in 50 pregnancies.

One study in Australia found that in a group of women who later developed endometriosis, one in 150 conceptions was ectopic before endometriosis developed. Among those later found to have endometriosis, the ectopic pregnancy rate was one in 60 pregnancies. This might suggest that ectopic pregnancy is more common in women with endometriosis. However, many different factors have been linked with ectopic pregnancy, including:

- abnormal tubal motility
- increased stickiness of tubal fluids
- pelvic inflammatory disease
- use of progestogen contraceptives
- use of the contraceptive coil
- previous abdominal surgery with adhesions
- tubal surgery for infertility
- reversal of female sterilisation.

There is no real evidence that ectopic pregnancy occurs with any greater frequency in women with endometriosis.

· *Symptoms* ·

Most ectopics are discovered in the first two months of development;

signs include pain and vaginal bleeding. In 80 per cent of cases, a period has already been missed, although in 20 per cent uterine bleeding makes it appear as if menstruation is continuing as usual.

As the fertilised egg starts to develop, the placenta burrows into surrounding tissues (e.g. thin Fallopian tube wall) rather than into spongy endometrium. The developing embryo becomes surrounded by a fluid-filled membrane to form a gestation sac.

Symptoms depend on the site of implantation. The wall of the inner two-thirds of the Fallopian tube (nearest the womb) is thin and less stretchy. As the early gestation sac swells, it dilates the tube to cause stretch pains and often triggers unexpected vaginal bleeding.

In this site, early rupture will occur within four to eight weeks of pregnancy if diagnosis is not made in time.

If the ectopic pregnancy is implanted in the outer, dilated end of the Fallopian tube symptoms tend to occur four weeks later (rupture at eight to twelve weeks of pregnancy) as the Fallopian tube walls here are wider apart and more stretchy. Blood may escape out into the abdominal cavity rather than down through the vagina, and the only symptom may be a dull, vague, intermittent ache to one side in the lower abdomen.

Usually, once bleeding occurs, the developing embryo dies. Continued bleeding causes swelling of the gestation sac and the Fallopian tube fills with blood to form what is known as a haematosalpynx.

Throughout the ectopic pregnancy, hormones secreted by the developing placenta have a partial effect on the endometrial lining of the womb. This swells up and undergoes a pregnancy reaction (decidualisation). Once the placenta dies, this is usually shed in pieces to cause some of the irregular bleeding that is a symptom of ectopic pregnancy.

Besides bleeding, other signs of an ecoptic pregnancy include:

- grumbling abdominal discomfort, occasional fainting, irregular vaginal bleeding or blood-stained discharge
- sudden abdominal pain and collapse
- pelvic pain plus a boggy swelling on examination
- advanced abdominal pregnancy with a normal-sized womb.

· *Diagnosis* ·

Ectopic pregnancy can be very difficult to diagnose clinically. The doctor may find tenderness in the lower abdomen to one side and a suggestion of a mass. Sometimes, however, confusion is caused when the tenderness is found to be on the opposite side to where the ectopic pregnancy is eventually found.

Internal examination can be just as unhelpful, but tenderness and a suggestion of a boggy mass are often detected to one side of the cervix.

If an ectopic pregnancy is suspected, you will probably have an ultra-sensitive pregnancy test and an ultrasound scan.

· *Pregnancy tests* ·

As the placenta develops, it secretes a hormone called human chorionic gonadotrophic hormone (hCG). This can now be detected in the blood within 48 hours after conception and in the urine within 72 hours of conception. If the pregnancy test is positive, the next step is to rule out a normal uterine pregnancy using ultrasound. If a gestation sac or a beating heart are seen in the womb, it makes an ectopic pregnancy extremely unlikely.

· *Ultrasound scans* ·

Two types of ultrasound scan are available: the familiar abdominal scan and the newer trans-vaginal scan.

With abdominal ultrasound, a full bladder is needed to help the operator orientate the probe and identify pelvic structures. It is unlikely that a gestation sac of an ectopic pregnancy would be visible before eight weeks of development.

Trans-vaginal ultrasound involves gently inserting a finger-shaped probe into the vagina. This technique is more accurate and can identify a developing yolk sac in the womb at five weeks of pregnancy, whether or not the bladder is full. There is one possible catch: if an ectopic pregnancy is present, the normal endometrium will be thickened by pregnancy hormones and show up as a false gestation sac in the womb.

Using trans-vaginal ultrasound, attempts can also be made to find the ectopic pregnancy within a Fallopian tube. It helps to identify the corpus luteum (see page 9) first, as in 90 per cent of cases, the ectopic pregnancy will develop on the same side.

The ultrasound appearance of an ectopic pregnancy varies, but it often looks like a thick ring known as the bagel sign! The gestation sac forms a black circle which is surrounded by a thickened ring of tissue. Sometimes an embryo or a beating heart is seen but this occurs only if the pregnancy is advanced.

Using high-quality trans-vaginal ultrasound, an ectopic pregnancy should be diagnosed in 90 per cent of cases where it is present.

Future diagnostic tests now being researched involve detecting increased blood flow to the area of ectopic pregnancy.

· *Treatment* ·

The treatment of an ectopic pregnancy is changing rapidly. Earlier and earlier diagnosis is possible due to sensitive pregnancy tests and the availability of trans-vaginal ultrasound.

Research suggests that in 50 per cent of cases where hCG levels are relatively low (less than 2,000 mIU/ml), the ectopic pregnancy will resolve on its own – either through spontaneous miscarriage or through natural reabsorption.

In health centres with advanced experience and technology, the decision to operate will depend on the ultrasound findings revealing the blood level of hCG. Surgery may be postponed while the woman is given repeat scans and a series of blood tests to watch which way hCG levels go. If the pregnancy resolves, the woman is spared surgery.

In some cases, the ectopic gestation sac has been injected with chemicals (methotrexate and 50 per cent dextrose solution) to kill it. The injection is made through the vagina using ultrasound control and is not yet widely available.

New techniques currently under research involve the use of tiny laser fibres inserted through needles to remove ectopic tissues under ultrasound control.

Surgical removal of the ectopic pregnancy is vital; otherwise it may rupture the tube, causing severe haemorrhage.

Diagnostic laparoscopy is performed first to confirm the ectopic pregnancy. Occasionally the embryo is removed using laparoscopic techniques, but most surgeons proceed to full laparotomy.

In early pregnancy, it is sometimes possible to slit open the Fallopian tube and gently squeeze out the products of conception. The surgeon may then repair the damaged tube using microsurgical techniques. Because damage increases the risk of a future ectopic pregnancy, many doctors prefer to remove the tube in its entirety. This is essential if rupture has already occurred. The surgeon clamps off the bleeding area, then removes the Fallopian tube, trying to save the ovary.

Signs of rupture include sudden abdominal pain, collapse, low blood pressure (shock) and a rigid, tender abdomen. Internal haemorrhage must be stemmed as soon as possible. Laparotomy will be done immediately without waiting for tests other than a blood count and cross-matching of blood for transfusion.

· *Future fertility* ·

It is still possible to have a normal pregnancy with only one Fallopian tube, although conception usually takes longer. This is because pregnancy can be successful only when ovulation occurs in the ovary on the unaffected side. Women with two damaged Fallopian tubes may successfully undergo *in vitro* fertilisation.

17

MISCARRIAGE

Miscarriage (also known as a spontaneous abortion) is defined as the failure of pregnancy before the 24th week of gestation. After this time, the sad event of fetal death is classified as a stillbirth.

Miscarriage is very common. Some studies suggest that up to 80 per cent of newly fertilised eggs (zygotes) fail to implant in the endometrium. This is known as pre-implantation wastage and occurs before conception is medically or legally recognised.

Of those zygotes that do successfully implant and start to produce a placenta, around 30 per cent miscarry – most before the mother is even aware that she is pregnant. The next period may be slightly later, and slightly heavier than usual, but that is all.

Of those pregnancies that are recognised as such by the mother, around 15 per cent fail to continue beyond the first five months of development. Twice as many will threaten to miscarry, with spotting of blood and cramp-like abdominal pains.

· *Endometriosis and miscarriage* ·

Some early studies seemed to show that miscarriage is up to three times more common in women with endometriosis than in the population at large. Rates as high as 49 per cent have been quoted – mostly within the first 12 weeks of pregnancy. Further studies suggested that this rate dropped significantly to around 8 per cent after surgical treatment.

More recently, however, the association between endometriosis and miscarriage has proved controversial. It is now generally agreed that there is no real evidence to suggest that miscarriage is more common in women with endometriosis. If it is, many researchers feel it is due to other factors, the most important of which is the woman's previous obstetric history, rather than the presence of endometriosis.

Among those who do believe endometriosis is linked with miscarriage, the most popular mechanism is thought to be inadequate progesterone levels (luteal defects) which are unable to prevent endometrial shedding (see page 9).

Factors linked with increased risk of miscarriage

Factors known to increase the risk of miscarriage in any woman include:

● Genetic abnormalities of the sperm or egg; these are mostly one-off reproductive accidents and occur in up to 60 per cent of recognised miscarriages, 5 per cent of stillbirths and 0.5 per cent of all live births.

● Nutritional deficiency, especially of folate (folic acid), vitamin B12, essential fatty acids, calcium, magnesium and zinc. Lack of these interferes with cell division and chromosome replication, a process occurring at a tremendous rate during fetal development.

● Smoking – women who smoke have a 27 per cent higher chance of suffering a miscarriage than non-smokers. Even passive smoking, especially where the mother lives with a smoker, has been linked with 4,000 miscarriages per year in the UK.

● Bacterial or viral infections such as rubella, chlamydia, anaerobic vaginosis or cytomegalovirus can result in miscarriage or congenital deformity if contracted during pregnancy. Other infections, such as influenza, pneumonia and appendicitis, can also trigger miscarriage, especially during the first three months of pregnancy. This is thought to be a protective mechanism as the mother's immune system is naturally depressed during pregnancy, decreasing her chance of fighting off the infection.

● Pre-existing disease in the mother, such as diabetes mellitus, high blood pressure, thyroid problems, epilepsy and anaemia, increase the risk of miscarriage if not carefully monitored and controlled.

● Auto-immune disease – especially systemic lupus erythematosus (SLE). In these conditions, the body makes antibodies against normal body structures which may attack the placenta or fetus as well. SLE is the auto-immune disease most usually linked with miscarriage. Among sufferers, 25 per cent have difficulty carrying pregnancy to term. Women with SLE tend to have high levels of anti-phospholipid antibody, aimed against cell membranes. These antibodies are also present in 15 per cent of women suffering a miscarriage for no known cause and who do not have SLE.

● Anatomical abnormalities of the female genital tract, such as a split (septate) uterus with two cavities, a double uterus or an incompetent cervix, can all result in miscarriage. These are relatively uncommon, with an incidence of around 1 in 700 women. An incompetent cervix is too weak to hold the womb closed after the third month of pregnancy. The problem is easily overcome by inserting a strong stitch around the cervix to hold it closed artifically. This stitch must be removed at around 37 weeks' gestation, or earlier if labour is premature.

● Immunological incompatibility between the fetus and the mother.

- Altered blood clotting mechanisms. As the developing pregnancy burrows into the uterus, slight bleeding occurs. A fine balance between local chemicals encouraging blood to clot and those causing clots to dissolve is set up. Altered blood-clotting mechanisms seem to be a common feature among women who suffer recurrent miscarriages.
- The use of drugs, including alcohol. Many of these are linked with early miscarriage or fetal abnormality. Only essential, prescribed drugs should be continued during pregnancy.
- New research is currently investigating a possible link between high levels of leutinising hormone (LH) and miscarriage.

· *Recurrent miscarriage* ·

In 95 per cent of cases, a single miscarriage is due to a non-recurring cause and there is an excellent chance of a future pregnancy continuing to term.

In most cases, a woman who has suffered two consecutive miscarriages has a 70 per cent chance of a future pregnancy's continuing to successful delivery of a child.

Recurrent miscarriage is diagnosed once three consecutive pregnancies have ended in spontaneous abortion. This affects around 1 in 200 pregnancies.

Tests are done to look for nutrient deficiencies, toxins, fetal, structural or genetic abnormalities, maternal uterine or cervical abnormalities, maternal systemic illnesses and immunological incompatibilities.

In 5 per cent of couples, an abnormal chromosome pattern is found in one partner which means they are unlikely successfully to produce a child. Genetic analysis and counselling is therefore an important part of the investigative process when recurrent miscarriage occurs.

There is some good news, however. Even women who have suffered from six or more miscarriages still have a 50 per cent chance of a future successful pregnancy, unless a specific, recurring abnormality is diagnosed.

18

FIBROIDS

The popular term, 'fibroid' is a bit of a misnomer as fibroids contain very little fibrous tissue. They are more properly known as *leiomyomas*. Like *endometriosis*, leiomyoma is a word that comes from the ancient Greek:

- *leios* is Greek for 'smooth',
- *myos* is Greek for 'muscle',
- *-oma* is a suffix meaning a growth or tumour.

A leiomyoma is therefore a benign (non-cancerous) tumour made up of smooth muscle fibres. These muscular knots also contain some framework cells (connective tissue) and can form in any muscle in the body. The most common site is in the muscle of the uterine wall. Other words that are sometimes used to describe a fibroid are 'myoma' (singular), 'myomata' (plural) and 'fibromyoma' (plural 'fibromyomata').

Although a fibroid is a tumour, it is a benign or non-cancerous growth. It is made up of cells that have the same structure as other cells in the type of tissue from which it has arisen. The nucleus of a fibroid cell looks normal, but for some reason the cells continue to multiply in an ordered, controlled fashion to form a lump. This presses on surrounding cells to squash them and form a surrounding capsule. Benign tumours do not invade surrounding tissues, nor can they spread throughout the body to form secondary tumours.

· *How common are fibroids?* ·

Fibroids are the commonest gynaecological condition – in fact, they are the commonest tumour in the human body. They are seen most frequently between the ages of 35 and 45. One in five women over the age of 30 and one in three women over the age of 35 are affected. They seldom occur before the age of 20 and never develop for the first time after the menopause. Once the menopause occurs, fibroid growth ceases and the tumours tend to regress, although hormone replacement therapy can sometimes reactivate and stimulate their growth.

In European women, fibroids seem to be most common in those who have not had children or who are relatively subfertile.

In women of Afro-American descent, fibroids seem to be more common at a younger age, often occurring in the late teens or early 20s, despite normal fertility.

· *The normal uterine wall* ·

The non-pregnant uterus is a pear-shaped, thick-walled, hollow muscle lying in the centre of the pelvis. It measures up to 10cm long and 5cm wide and its wall is approximately 3cm thick. It weighs around 60–90g and is made up of two layers:

- the inner lining (endometrium)
- the middle smooth muscle coat (myometrium).

The back wall of the uterus and the upper body (fundus) are covered by the peritoneal membrane which lines the floor of the pelvic cavity. The development of the womb is discussed on page 5.

The muscle that makes up the myometrium consists of millions of bundles of muscle fibres that form a stretchy mesh. Collagen fibres snake through this mesh to form a strong framework, and a rich blood supply feeds both the muscle and the inner endometrial lining.

Uterine muscle looks smooth when examined under a microscope and is therefore called smooth muscle. In contrast, skeletal muscle (such as biceps) looks striped when examined under a microscope; this type of muscle is called striated muscle.

Smooth and striated muscles have different roles in the body. Striated muscle tends to be under our voluntary control (e.g. arm movements) while smooth muscles are concerned with involuntary movements such as the muscular wave-like activity that propels food through the gut (peristalsis) and the muscular contractions of the womb during menstruation, orgasm and childbirth.

· *How fibroids form* ·

A fibroid starts off as a tiny whorl of spindle-shaped muscle cells. These come together to form an interlacing bundle similar to a fingerprint whorl. The muscle cells in this small fibroid continue to grow abnormally, at a faster rate than surrounding muscle fibres, to form a solid, rubbery ball of cells. This seedling fibroid slowly expands to compress normal muscle fibres surrounding it. This results in formation of a thickened, false capsule around it. The presence of this false capsule allows a surgeon to distinguish a fibroid from an adenomyoma – the fibroid-like gland and muscle cell swelling that can occur in adenomyosis (see page 34) – which has no capsule.

Small tumours consist purely of muscle fibres, although larger tumours also contain some gristly fibrous tissue.

· *What a fibroid looks like* ·

Imagine a knot in a plank of wood; this is similar to the appearance of a fibroid – a muscular knot surrounded by the smooth muscle of the uterus.

The muscle of the womb itself is a pinkish grey. If a fibroid is cut in half, it looks like a hard, round, white ball of cells in which a whorled structure can be made out. On examination under a microscope, the long spindle-shaped muscle cells are found to form interlacing bundles, rather like the scalloped plasterwork that was popular in the 1970s.

Fibroids vary in size and can be as small as a pea or as large as a grapefruit. They can be single, but are more often multiple – the maximum number removed from one patient was 200.

Fibroid size tends to be compared to the size of a pregnant uterus. If the diameter and volume of a fibroid enlarges the womb to the size of a 12-week pregnancy, it is considered large. In extreme cases, a fibroid can mimic the size of 20-week fetus and one fibroid was found that weighed over 11kg.

Fibroids can be found in any part of the uterus, although 95 per cent arise in the body of the uterus and only 5 per cent in the cervix. The following types are recognised:

- submucosal (or sub-endometrial) – a tumour just beneath the endometrium that bulges into the womb cavity
- fibroid polyp – a tumour that develops a stalk (pedicle) to dangle into the uterine cavity, rather like the clapper of a bell; this is also called a pedunculated fibroid
- intramural – a fibroid that forms in the middle of the uterine wall to cause a localised thickening
- subserous (sub-peritoneal) – a fibroid that forms near the outer surface of the uterus to bulge into the pelvic cavity
- subserous polyp – a fibroid covered in peritoneal membrane which develops a pedicle and hangs off the outer uterine wall
- intraligamentary – a fibroid that extends sideways between the two leaves of the broad ligament suspending the uterus in the pelvis
- cervical – a fibroid that forms in the cervix; these can sometimes grow to such a size that the uterus is pushed up on top of the tumour, likened to the 'lantern on the dome of St Paul's'.

A large fibroid can form a mechanical distortion that protrudes into the uterus and alters the shape of the cavity, compresses or blocks the Fallopian tubes and changes the anatomical relationship between the Fallopian tubes and the ovaries.

· *What causes fibroids?* ·

The cause of fibroids is unknown, but they are thought to represent an abnormal growth response of uterine smooth muscle cells to the female hormone, oestrogen.

Oestrogen has a proliferative growth effect on the endometrium and breasts and also maintains the juicy, youthful state of other tissues in the reproductive tract (see page X). If oestrogen is withdrawn (at the menopause, for example) reproductive tissues, including the muscle of the uterine wall, start to wither. This implies that oestrogen has a growth-stimulating effect on uterine smooth muscle. It is thought that fibroids form when smooth muscle cells become oversensitive to this oestrogen effect. Although it is difficult to understand why such a response is localised to certain parts of the uterine wall, this theory is supported by the fact that fibroids tend to enlarge in women with an unusually high oestrogen state, such as:

- some women on the oral contraceptive pill
- women who are pregnant
- some women who are on HRT
- women who are very overweight, because their fatty tissues can make oestrogen from other sex hormones in the body.

Fibroids can also occur in women who show other signs of high oestrogen levels unbalanced by the other female hormone, progesterone. This happens in women who regularly fail to ovulate during their menstrual cycle.

Decreased oestrogen levels after the menopause usually cause fibroids to shrink. They may therefore be linked to some sort of common, localised change in oestrogen receptors present on the outer surface of a single muscle cell. As this cell divides and multiplies to form identical cells with identical over-sensitive oestrogen receptors, it might provide a mechanism for fibroid formation and growth.

Drugs that lower oestrogen levels (some of which are used to treat endometriosis) have proved helpful in shrinking fibroids.

Some doctors believe that fibroids may be triggered by pelvic congestion, as can occur in some women with premenstrual syndrome. Although this isn't proved, it seems that regular pelvic exercises that stimulate pelvic blood flow can shrink fibroids in some cases (see page 168).

· *Symptoms* ·

In many cases, fibroids cause no symptoms at all, especially if they are small. Even if a fibroid is large, if it does not press on surrounding organs (such as the bladder) or protrude into the cavity of the womb, it may go undetected. In 50 per cent of cases, women with fibroids develop symptoms that are bad enough to need medical help.

Heavy periods

One-third of women with fibroids suffer from abnormal bleeding, usually during menstruation but occasionally between periods also. Heavy periods can occur even with small or only moderately sized tumours.

The commonest cause of heavy bleeding is a submucosal fibroid. This protrudes into the uterine cavity to enlarge the surface area of the endometrium – sometimes by as much as 15 times. This means there is more endometrium to shed during a menstrual period and heavy bleeding (menorrhagia) results.

The presence of a large muscular growth in the uterine wall also increases the number and size of blood vessels supplying the womb, making a heavy period more likely.

Another factor that can make periods particularly heavy in women with fibroids is that they are linked with high oestrogen levels. Oestrogen stimulates the lining of the womb and causes it to proliferate, so there is more tissue to shed each month.

If a fibroid extends into the middle of the uterine wall (intramural fibroid), it will interfere with the normal, ordered contraction of the uterine muscle during a period. This may prevent the closing off of bleeding arteries (which may already be larger than normal) after the outer endometrial layer is shed, so that the period continues longer and is heavier than usual. It may also result in muscular cramping pains to produce painful periods.

Heavy bleeding may include large clots, and if you lose too much blood you may develop iron-deficiency anaemia over several months. Depending on how bad it is, anaemia can cause:

- pallor
- headache
- tiredness
- faintness
- dizziness
- weakness
- shortness of breath
- rapid pulse
- palpitations
- swollen ankles
- spoon-shaped nails (in long-term iron deficiency)
- sore tongue
- cracks at corners of the mouth

- increased susceptibility to infections
- chest pains (angina)
- pains in calves on walking.

In extreme cases, large fibroids may cause a a life-threatening haemorrhage.

If you have heavy periods, this does not necessarily mean that you have a fibroid. The excessive bleeding could have many other causes, including:

- hormonal imbalances and lack of ovulation
- endometriosis
- polyps
- pregnancy
- pelvic infection
- intra-uterine contraceptive device (IUCD – coil)
- endometrial or ovarian cancer
- thyroid or pituitary gland problems
- clotting disorders.

Painful periods

During menstruation, fibroids interfere with the normal, ordered contractions of the womb, which can trigger painful, prolonged cramps. If the fibroid hangs into the uterine cavity on a stalk it may trigger local irritation and uterine contractions as the womb tries to expel it. This can cause intermittent cramping pains, rather like a mini-labour, especially during a period. This may also occur between periods and can be associated with spotting of blood.

Painful sex

Although it is unusual for fibroids to cause painful intercourse, some women do seem to be affected. They can suffer pain on deep penetration during intercourse (deep dyspareunia) because an enlarged uterus, or a subserous fibroid on its outer wall, is pushed against an ovary. The ovaries are just as tender as the male testicles but this problem is usually noticed only in certain sexual positions, and it is worth experimenting to find a position that is pain-free for you.

During orgasm, the womb undergoes a series of contractions that contribute to the wave-like sensations felt. Sometimes a fibroid in the uterine wall can cause unpleasant sensations during orgasm which may be perceived as painful.

Rarely, pain during sex is due to a polyp fibroid that has been partially expelled from the womb cavity and has become stuck in the cervical canal. This can cause pain and spotting throughout the menstrual cycle, but especially when making love.

Even more rarely, a polyp fibroid can be expelled from the womb into the vagina, but remain attached on the end of its stalk. It can then enlarge at the top of the vagina, which will also cause pain and bleeding during sex. This is easily noticed by a doctor performing an internal examination and visual inspection of the cervix, for example when taking a smear.

Swelling

Many women with fibroids suffer from sensations of fullness, pressure pain and dragging sensations. This is most common with slowly enlarging intramural or subserosal fibroids (see page 128).

If the fibroids are large or multiple, the uterus will be enlarged to several times its normal size. This may cause a sensation of bloating, abdominal swelling and the presence of a heavy lump in the pelvis. A woman may have an unpleasant sensation of something coming down if the uterus starts to prolapse.

If the fibroid presses against pelvic veins, the circulation will be compromised and the veins lower down from the blockage may become engorged. This can lead to aching in the lower limbs, swollen legs, varicose veins and haemorrhoids (piles).

Urinary and bowel symptoms

Sometimes pressure from a fibroid can cause bladder or bowel symptoms. A large frontal fibroid that presses on the bladder may reduce urinary capacity or cause symptoms of irritation, along with one or more of the following:

- frequent need to urinate
- urgency (having to rush to the loo)
- hesitancy (having to strain to start)
- painful spasm on urination
- passing only small amounts of urine.

These symptoms are often mistaken for cystitis.

Similarly, if the fibroid is positioned at the back of the uterus, it may press on the rectum to cause:

- a sensation of a lump in the rectum
- a frequent urge to open the bowels
- spasm of the rectum (tenesmus)
- constipation.

· *Always tell your doctor* ·

Occasionally, a large fibroid presses on pelvic veins that bring blood up from the legs or from the anal region. This interference with blood supply can sometimes trigger varicose veins or piles.

If you notice any of the above symptoms (unusual bleeding, swelling, spotting between periods, painful sex, bowel or bladder problems) you should tell your doctor straight away. Besides indicating fibroids, they can also be signs of other conditions which may need urgent medical treatment.

· *Complications* ·

Fibroids are associated with a few complications:

- They may cause recurrent miscarriage due to gross distortion of the womb cavity.
- Very rarely, a pedunculated fibroid may twist around on its stalk to cut off its blood supply (torsion); this usually causes severe low abdominal pain, shock and vomiting. Usually, the symptoms are bad enough for the sufferer to be admitted to hospital with acute abdominal pain, and the twisted fibroid is removed surgically. Occasionally, torsion causes few symptoms and the diagnosis is not made. The fibroid may then die and wither away, become infected or pick up another blood supply from nearby adhesions so that it acts rather like a parasite, becoming detached and independent of the uterus.
- Also, rarely, a large fibroid may become stuck in the pelvis (impacted) during menstruation or pregnancy, blocking off the passage of urine (acute retention).

· *Degeneration* ·

If a fibroid continues to grow, the arteries and veins supplying the uterine muscle enlarge considerably (hypertrophy) to supply an ever-increasing volume of blood. Eventually, however, the tumours may outgrow their blood supply, which results in several different patterns of degeneration:

- atrophy – the natural regression of a fibroid after oestrogen is withdrawn at the menopause
- hyaline degeneration – found in most large fibroids; the central cells die due to lack of nutrients and oxygen to form a glassy, pink substance similar to transparent cartilage, which lacks any cells
- cystic degeneration – the next stage on from hyaline change, with central liquefaction of the tumour
- calcareous degeneration – deposition of calcium, especially in larger fibroids in older women; on an X-ray this resembles stones
- red degeneration – sudden blockage of blood supply so that fibroid

tissues die (infarct). If this occurs, it is often during pregnancy. The tumour changes by swelling, becoming red in colour and softening, usually with severe abdominal pain. There is a risk of miscarriage or premature labour as red degeneration can trigger uterine contraction. Drugs can be given to stop contractions and the fibroid will shrink down once the baby is born

- malignant degeneration – conversion of a benign fibroid tumour into a malignant cancer known as a sarcoma; although sarcoma is rare in fibroids (one in every 200) the fact that fibroids are so common means that this is the most frequently encountered type of womb sarcoma. It is usually discovered unexpectedly at operation.

· *Fibroids and fertility* ·

Fibroids are not a major cause of subfertility, but some doctors estimate they are associated with 5 per cent of cases. This may simply be because by the time fibroids have developed, during the late 30s and early 40s, fertility has naturally decreased anyway. Fibroids can cause mechanical problems with the womb, however, and it is possible that these changes are linked with subfertility:

- disruption of the endometrial lining
- distortion of the normal relationship between the ovary and Fallopian tube
- blockage of the bottom end of a Fallopian tube where it passes through the uterine muscle to open into the uterine cavity
- blockage of the cervix canal so that sperm cannot swim through as easily
- distortion of the endometrium so that implantation of a fertilised egg is interfered with.

Large fibroids are associated with an increased risk of miscarriage due to mechanical distortion, red degeneration and competing with the blood flow that is needed to nourish a pregnancy.

Fibroids may not be suspected before pregnancy. Because they make the womb seem much larger they can make the pregnancy seem more advanced than it really is, or cause suspicion of twins. Once a routine ultrasound scan is performed to check pregnancy dates and fetal development (around 16–18 weeks' pregnancy) the correct diagnosis will be made.

A large fibroid can interfere with childbirth, especially if it grows near the cervical entrance. This is uncommon, as usually the fibroid rides up higher into the uterus as the surrounding muscle is stretched. Occasionally, however, an elective Caesarean section may be recommended if the fibroid stops the baby's head from settling low in the pelvis or if it encourages a breech (bottom first) presentation.

19

DIAGNOSIS OF FIBROIDS

Symptomless fibroids often remain undetected but may be picked up on a routine internal examination or on ultrasound during early pregnancy. Otherwise, fibroids come to light once they start causing symptoms, such as those previously described (see page 129). If uterine distortion is pronounced, fibroids may be diagnosed during investigation for recurrent miscarriage or subfertility.

· *Abdominal examination* ·

A uterus that is enlarged by the presence of a fibroid to the size of a 12-week pregnancy can usually be felt by examining the abdomen. The fibroid will be detected arising above the brim of the pelvic bone, usually in the centre but occasionally off to one side. It can be difficult to tell whether the lump is part of the uterus, ovaries, or even bowel, so an internal examination is essential.

A diagnosis of fibroids based on an abdominal and pelvic examination is correct 85 per cent of the time. There is still room for error, however, as conditions such as endometriomas, tumours, adenomyomas, bowel masses, pelvic inflammatory disease, adhesions or even normal pregnancy can easily be mistaken for fibroids.

· *Internal examination* ·

During an internal examination, the doctor performs a bimanual assessment of the womb. One hand is placed on the abdomen above the pubic bone, while two fingers of the other hand are gently inserted into the vagina. By pressing upwards on the cervix, the doctor tries to feel the top of the uterus (fundus) with the hand resting on your abdomen. If the fundus can be felt, this implies that the womb is enlarged and bulky. Sometimes a fibroid can easily be detected as a smooth, firm lump arising either in the midline or off to one side. Having felt a lump, the doctor then needs to work out if it arises from the uterus or elsewhere, such as an ovary. Generally, by moving the cervix the doctor can work out whether the lump moves in co-ordination with the cervix (and is therefore part of the womb), or if it moves separately from the cervix (and may be part of the ovary).

· *Blood tests* ·

A few blood tests are helpful in diagnosing fibroids. A full blood count will show whether you have iron-deficiency anaemia or not. At least 70 per cent of women who regularly lose over 80ml of blood per period (the definition of menorrhagia) will have some degree of anaemia. The others will have iron deficiency insufficient to lower the haemoglobin level but sufficient to lower levels of a blood chemical, ferritin. Blood ferritin levels reflect the amount of stored iron in your body and should therefore be measured as well.

An under- or overactive thyroid can cause irregular, heavy periods. Blood tests are therefore often carried out to assess thyroid function.

If you have bowel or bladder symptoms, blood tests to assess kidney and liver function may be done routinely.

· *Ultrasound* ·

Ultrasound is the most useful test for diagnosing fibroids. These tumours have a characteristic appearance that enable them to be distinguished from other pelvic cysts and their diameter and volume can be accurately measured. (Ultrasound is described more fully on page 52.)

It is important that a doctor examine you internally before referring you for ultrasound. In some cases, large ovarian cysts have been missed because they were in the abdominal cavity rather than the pelvis.

· *Endometrial biopsy* ·

If you have heavy periods, or notice spotting of blood, your doctor may want to obtain a sample of endometrial tissue for examination under a microscope.

There are three main ways of doing this:

- using a sampling device to take a 'blind' biopsy sample
- using a telescopic viewing device (hysteroscopy) and taking a biopsy under visual control
- a full dilation and curettage (D&C or scrape).

In women over the age of 40, endometrial biopsy is usually performed to exclude more serious causes of heavy bleeding such as endometrial infection, excessive stimulation by oestrogen hormone (cystic hyperplasia – a pre-cancerous condition) and endometrial cancer itself. It may also indicate whether an otherwise healthy endometrium seems excessively thick.

In women under the age of 40 biopsy is not always performed, as endometrial cancer is uncommon below this age. Many doctors consider endometrial sampling unnecessary unless you have a history of irregular bleeding or progressive bleeding that does not respond to drug treatment. Biopsy may be deferred unless your bleeding is excessively heavy or associated with spotting between periods or after sex.

Suction biopsy is a relatively easy procedure that can be performed in a GP surgery (not yet common) or in an outpatient clinic. It is similar to having an intrauterine contraceptive device fitted and you do not need an anaesthetic.

The doctor inserts a vaginal speculum and gently introduces a special, narrow biopsy rod into the uterus through the cervical canal. By manipulating the device, and applying light suction, he or she can attract a small 1–2 cm long strip of superficial endometrium into the pipette and then slice it off by activating a blade. This procedure is performed 'blind' and there is a small risk that it may miss an endometrial lesion, such as a polyp, that is present elsewhere in the uterus and so produce a misleadingly normal biopsy. In general, however, the risk of missing an endometrial cancer is small. The advantage of this simple biopsy technique is that it does not entail a general anaesthetic. The disadvantage is that it will not diagnose endometrial polyps or submucous fibroids.

Hysteroscopy is the investigation of choice of many gynaecologists, especially for women over the age of 45 who have irregular, heavy, painful periods or spotting between periods or after sex.

You may be given a choice between a local anaesthetic (injected into the cervix) or a light, general anaesthetic. It is usually performed as an outpatient procedure. So-called 'one-stop clinics' are now in place, allowing women a full assessment including pelvic ultrasound, hysteroscopy, biopsy and blood tests to measure haemoglobin and thyroid function.

First, the vagina is cleansed with an antiseptic, then the cervical canal is gently dilated (if necessary) by passing a series of rods of gradually increasing diameter. A telescopic viewing device (hysteroscope), about 1cm wide, is then inserted so that the surgeon can carefully examine the entire endometrial lining of your womb. This has several channels in it, one for looking down, one for a fibre-optic light, one for passing through fluid or gas (to separate the walls of the womb and to wash away blood or parings) plus a channel for fine biopsy or cauterising instruments.

A fibroid bulging into the endometrial cavity is easily seen at hysteroscopy, as are any endometrial polyps or other abnormal lesions. The surgeon can pick the spots where he or she wants to take a biopsy under direct visual control. Lesions such as endometrial polyps or fibroid polyps can also be removed for examination.

D&C was once a common procedure used in the UK both to investigate and to treat heavy, painful periods. In 1993, a study showed that D&C was performed six times more often in the UK than in the US, although hysterectomy rates are much higher in the States.

D&C is now becoming increasingly unpopular and is often dismissed as diagnostically inaccurate and therapeutically ineffective. It also carries some risks such as trauma and inadvertent perforation and post-operative infection. Nevertheless, D&C may still be indicated in some women, especially where hysteroscopy is not available.

D&C involves a light general anaesthetic (although it can be performed under a local) and is generally performed on an outpatient basis.

The surgeon will first examine you fully under anaesthetic to assess the size and shape of your womb. The cervical canal will then be gently dilated by passing through it a series of metal rods, each slightly wider than the last. The surgeon will also attach a long clip to the cervix to hold the womb steady.

Next, the surgeon inserts a metal instrument with a spoon-like scrape on the end and systematically scrapes away the outer layer of the womb lining (the part that is usually shed during a period). Samples of the scrapings are then sent for analysis under a microscope.

Following a D&C you will have light bleeding and sometimes mild period-like pains for a few days. You should wear sanitary towels to catch this light flow rather than tampons, to minimise the risk of infection in the raw endometrial tissues after the operation. The vagina is full of bacteria, and infection cannot always be prevented. If you notice increasing pain, bleeding or an unpleasant-smelling discharge, tell your doctor straight away in case you need antibiotics.

Don't resume sexual relations until the bleeding or any discharge has settled down.

· *Other tests for fibroids* ·

If you have other symptoms such as spotting of blood, unidentified pelvic mass, swelling of legs, or bowel or bladder symptoms, you may have one or more additional tests:

- urinalysis (for blood and protein)
- intravenous pyelogram (IVP) to check your kidney function (see page 59)
- stool analysis to look for hidden blood
- a venogram – a dye test to show up your venous circulation
- CAT or MRI scans (see page 53).

If any doubt remains as to whether you have fibroids or another sort of pelvic tumour, laparoscopy and/or laparotomy may be necessary.

· *Treatment* ·

Small symptomless fibroids usually require no treatment. You will be regularly reassessed to ensure they are not growing too large and not causing undue problems during menstruation.

Once your fibroids cause serious symptoms or complications, treatment is required. This can be medical (drugs) or surgical.

· *The medical treatment of fibroids* ·

Prostaglandin inhibitors

Aspirin can be effective in relieving menstrual cramping pains. It works by stopping the production of hormone-like chemicals (prostaglandins – see page 38). Women with heavy, painful periods tend to have higher than normal concentrations of prostaglandins in their menstrual flow. This is thought to trigger inflammation and painful spasm of muscles in the uterus, to increase dilation and bleeding of endometrial blood vessels, and to interfere with normal blood-clotting mechanisms. Prostaglandins therefore have a large role to play in maintaining a prolonged, heavy, painful period. Treatment with aspirin-like drugs (also called non-steroidal anti-inflammatory drugs – NSAIDs) can sometimes dramatically improve menstrual symptoms by reducing pain, inflammation and blood loss. They can be taken throughout the period and are most effective if started one or two days before the period is due – especially if premenstrual pain is common.

As well as aspirin, stronger NSAIDs are available – some over the counter (e.g. ibuprofen) and some only on prescription (e.g. mefenamic acid, naproxen). They seem to be effective and reduce blood flow by up to 33 per cent.

Aspirin-like drugs can cause the following side effects (many of which are rare) in some people if taken long-term. Side effects are uncommon if the drugs are taken for only a few days during menstruation each month.

Possible side effects of aspirin-like drugs include:

- nausea
- diarrhoea
- indigestion (best taken after food)
- gastric bleeding (usually microscopic, but occasional haemorrhages)
- blood in the urine (haematuria)
- an asthma attack in asthmatics
- thinning of the blood (may be a desirable effect in some cases)
- allergic skin rashes or tissue swelling (angio-oedema)

- fluid retention
- blood disorders (e.g. low platelet count – rare)
- dizziness and confusion (in overdose)
- buzzing in ears (tinnitus) and deafness in overdose.

Aspirin-like drugs should not be taken, except under medical supervision by the following:

- pregnant women
- women who are breast-feeding
- children under the age of 12
- the elderly
- people with indigestion or active peptic ulcers
- people with a history of gastritis or peptic ulcers
- people with asthma
- people with heart, kidney or liver failure
- people with some metabolic diseases
- people with haemophilia or other bleeding disorders
- people with gout
- people taking warfarin
- people taking any other drugs, except with the doctor's permission.

Blood-clotting mediators

During menstruation, there is a fine balance between enzyme actions that trigger blood clotting and fibrinolytic enzymes that break clots down again (see page 11). If bleeding is heavy, clotting enzymes are overwhelmed and bleeding from the endometrium continues unchecked. Women with menorrhagia also seem to have excessive fibrinolytic (plasminogen) activity in their menstrual flow, which liquefies any clots that do manage to form. As a result, flooding occurs.

Drugs that have anti-fibrinolytic activity (e.g. tranexamic acid, epsilon-amino caproic acid) are sometimes prescribed to inhibit the excessive fibrinolytic activity to encourage early stemming of the blood flow. They are taken only during menstruation and seem to be effective, reducing blood flow by up to 50 per cent.

Although there was formerly concern that these drugs might trigger blood clots elsewhere in the body, they have now been shown to be safe in normal, healthy women even for long periods of time. They should not be taken by women with a history of blood-clotting disorders, however.

Ethamsylate is another haemostatic agent that helps to stop bleeding. It is thought to work by maintaining the integrity of capillary walls, thereby minimising bleeding from these tiny blood vessels. It also inhibits the action of prostaglandins and an enzyme, hyaluronidase, which is involved in tissue breakdown and inflammation during endometrial sloughing. Its use in menorrhagia is still experimental and as yet there are few studies to show how effective it is. It should not be taken by people with porphyria (a rare metabolic disorder).

Possible side effects of these drugs include:

- nausea
- vomiting
- headache
- diarrhoea
- giddiness
- allergic rashes
- blood clotting disease (thromboembolism).

Oral contraceptive pills (OCP)

Oral contraceptives are probably the first line of treatment in women who have small submucous fibroids with heavy, painful periods and who also want effective contraception. Although early formulations of the OCP, which contained high doses of oestrogen, were found to trigger sudden growth of pre-existing fibroids in some women and were also linked with red degeneration (see page 133), modern pill formulations are lower in dose and have been found beneficial in treating the menorrhagia of fibroids. Two major studies have shown that:

- fibroids are less common in users of low-oestrogen pills than in non-users
- those suffering from fibroids are less likely to need referral to hospital for investigation and treatment if the patient is on OCP
- the OCP almost always reduces heavy bleeding associated with fibroids.

The combined oral contraceptive pill (COCP) contains two synthetic hormones, an oestrogen and a progestogen. It is taken every day for 21 days, and then a 7-day pill-free interval occurs during which contraceptive protection is still provided.

The combined Pill inhibits secretion of follicle-stimulating hormone (FSH) and leutinising hormone (LH) by the pituitary gland. Without these, ovarian egg follicles do not start to mature each month and ovulation therefore stops. The Pill also has an effect on the endometrium and thins it down. As well as its contraceptive action of reducing the risk of fertilisation, this also reduces the volume of menstrual flow, even where the endometrial surface area is enlarged by a submucous fibroid.

If you have fibroids you will be put on a COCP that is predominantly progestogenic. You will need regular examinations, however, to ensure that the fibroid does not unexpectedly increase in size during the treatment.

The COCP makes blood more sticky by promoting the clumping together of blood cell fragments called platelets. These help blood to clot and seal small wounds and will also reduce the amount of blood lost during menstrual sloughing. Occasionally, the COCP can trigger abnormal blood clotting, and thrombosis can occur. These blood clots can break off and travel round the body to cause problems.

Smoking cigarettes greatly increases the risk of blood clotting so, once a female smoker reaches the age of 35, she should use another method of contraception – and this is the age at which fibroids are likely to become troublesome. You can continue with the COCP only if you do not smoke. It is now acceptable for women who don't smoke to use a new, low-dose, combined pill right up until they reach the menopause.

Possible side effects of the Pill include:
- nausea
- headache
- mood changes such as depression
- changes in sex drive (raised or lowered)
- lack of periods
- breakthrough bleeding between periods
- breast tenderness
- weight gain
- intolerance to contact lenses
- light-sensitive skin discolouration
- blood clots (less common in women with blood group O)
- high blood pressure
- stroke (rare)
- jaundice or other liver disease.

The COCP should not be taken by women who:
- are pregnant
- are breast-feeding
- are over 35 and who smoke
- have high blood pressure
- are obese
- have some complications of diabetes
- have coronary heart disease
- have severe migraine
- have gallstones
- have liver disease
- have otosclerosis (a type of impaired hearing)
- have porphyria (a rare metabolic disease)
- have undiagnosed, abnormal vaginal bleeding
- have a history of blood-clotting disorders
- have a history of certain problems during pregnancy (pruritis, pemphigoid gestationis, jaundice)

- have a history of hormone-dependent tumour (e.g. of the cervix or breast) unless under medical supervision.

Progestogens

Progestogens are often used to treat heavy menstrual bleeding, but they are unlikely to be of benefit unless menorrhagia is due to a relative progesterone deficiency (deficient luteal phase) which occurs in anovulatory cycles. If a deficient luteal phase is present, natural progesterone suppositories are the treatment of choice, not a synthetic progestogen. Nevertheless, a progestogen such as norethisterone is frequently prescribed from the 19th to the 26th day of the menstrual cycle.

Progestogens are best given in combination with an oestrogen (as a COCP) as their action in depleting the endometrium is most efficient if the endometrium has been primed with oestrogen beforehand.

Medicated intra-uterine contraceptive devices which release natural progesterone or a synthetic progestogen (levonorgestrel) have been shown to reduce blood loss substantially where a reliable method of contraception is needed. Once inserted, the device lasts for five years. These coils are not yet widely available, however, and may not be recommended in a woman with a large, fibroid uterus because of difficulties in insertion, risk of perforation and increased chance of the device being expelled from the uterus.

For more information on progestogens, see page 66.

Danazol

Danazol is sometimes used to treat fibroids on an experimental basis, though few trials have been carried out to discover just how effective it is. Even when used in relatively small doses (compared with those used to treat endometriosis) of 100–200mg per day, it reduces menstrual blood loss and bleeding becomes more regular. By reducing circulating levels of oestrogen hormone, danazol may shrink fibroid volume.

In one study of 155 patients with menorrhagia, 43 were found to have fibroids. After treatment with danazol, overall 82 per cent of the 155 women noted a return to their normal pattern of menstruation. The group that had fibroids were unfortunately not looked at separately to see if their response rate was the same, better or worse than that of the group in general.

For more information about danazol, see page 75.

Gestrinone

Gestrinone has an effect similar to that of danazol and, by reducing levels of circulating oestrogen hormone, has been shown to reduce the volume of fibroids. For information about gestrinone, see page 72.

GnRH analogues

GnRH analogues have recently been used experimentally to treat fibroids. By reducing circulating oestrogen levels and inducing a reversible, false menopause, they can shrink fibroids down. However, the drugs can be used for only six months and fibroids may regrow after treatment. For more information about GnRH analogues, see page 79.

· *The surgical treatment of fibroids* ·

Most women with fibroids never need to resort to surgery as their symptoms are non-severe or adequately controlled with drugs. In this case, a wait-and-see game is played, with regular internal examinations to ensure the uterus is not becoming too bulky.

If heavy, painful periods cause undue misery – in some cases a woman is bleeding for three weeks out of four – surgery may be the only option. This is especially likely if the uterus is enlarged to the size of a 16-week pregnancy or more.

If you hope to have more children, or cannot face the thought of a hysterectomy, your fibroids can be shelled out, leaving the uterus intact, during an operation called a myomectomy:

- *myoma* is Greek for 'fibroid',
- *-ectomy* is Greek for 'removal of'.

Myomectomy therefore means removal of fibroids. This is feasible only if your fibroids are easily accessible on the outer surface of the uterus. Submucous fibroids – often the cause of menorrhagia – are diffiicult to shell out because the surgeon can get at them only by cutting or tunnelling through the full thickness of the uterine wall. This obviously weakens the muscle, increases the risk of operative bleeding and may cause problems during future pregnancies.

Newly developed techniques using a hysteroscope have now made these submucous fibroids more easily and safely accessible via the vagina and uterine cavity. Lasers are also now used to obliterate fibroids.

If you have completed your family and if your fibroids are large, a hysterectomy may be suggested. If your fibroids are relatively small, surgical resection of the endometrium (leaving the muscle and fibroids behind) may be your best option. Occasionally, however, fibroids cause a spontaneous, massive haemorrhage and hysterectomy then becomes an emergency, life-saving procedure. These techniques are all discussed below.

Endometrial resection of submucous fibroids

Most cases of menorrhagia are associated with small or medium submucous fibroids (under the endometrium) that bulge into the uterine cavity, increasing its surface area. Using a hysteroscope (see page 137) a surgeon can remove these fibroids so that periods return to normal and fertility is preserved. This is usually done under general anaesthetic on an outpatient basis. Occasionally, a local anaesthetic (injected into the cervix) plus a sedative is used.

The technique is similar to that for a diagnostic hysteroscopy (see page 137). A laser beam is used via the hysteroscope to pare away individual small fibroids in slices. The laser can also be used to remove pedunculated fibroid polyps.

A similar procedure uses a hot cutting wire instead of a laser. The instrument used is called a resectoscope. The hot wire can cut and cauterise a submucous fibroid as easily as a laser beam and is a cheaper, less sophisticated option.

After resection of a fibroid, you will have a slight, watery, blood-stained discharge for a few days. This should be absorbed with a sanitary towel rather than a tampon to reduce the risk of infection ascending from the vagina. If you notice excessive bleeding, pain or a foul-smelling discharge, tell your doctor straight away. Normal sexual relations can usually resume after your next period has finished.

Myomectomy

Because fibroids are enclosed in a capsule formed from the squashing of surrounding tissues, they can be shelled out using the equivalent of a large corkscrew. This is an attractive option for younger women who do not want to face sterility. To minimise bleeding, you may be given drug treatments (e.g. danazol or GnRH agonists) to shrink your fibroids down before the operation.

Myomectomy is often technically more difficult than hysterectomy. It may not be possible if your fibroids are too big or too numerous or the uterus is too enlarged. It increases the risk of excessive bleeding and weakening or scarring of the uterus, which may cause problems with future pregnancies.

Myomectomy can be performed through a low abdominal (bikini-line) or vaginal incision, depending on the site of the fibroid(s) to be removed. Once the uterus is exposed, an astonishing number of fibroids are sometimes found – several dozen is not unusual. These range in size from small seedling tumours to growths weighing several kilograms.

Myomectomy is used to remove subserosal and intramural fibroids (see page 128). The surgeon carefully cuts into the surrounding fibroid capsule with a scalpel, laser or hot diathermy wire, being careful not to nick the fibroid itself, which would trigger bleeding. Sometimes the fibroid can be coaxed out by inserting a lever, such as the handle of the scalpel, into the capsule and shelling it out, rather like removing a broad bean from its pod. Alternatively, a large corkscrew can be twisted into the tumour so the surgeon can pull it out just like removing a cork from a bottle. To avoid making further incisions in the uterine wall, the surgeon then aims to enter other fibroid capsules through the defect left from the first fibroid removed. The skill of the surgeon lies in deciding where to place the incisions and when to tunnel through the space left by a previously shelled fibroid, to avoid excessive weakening of the uterine wall.

Fibroids have a rich blood supply and extensive shelling out may cause massive haemorrhage. The surgeon will usually stem this with diathermy (hot electro-cautery) although a laser may sometimes be available (see below). Bleeding arteries can be pinched off and tied or drugs injected into the fibroid capsule to trigger clotting.

Subserosal pedunculated fibroids are more easily dealt with by simply clamping off the stalk of the fibroid, tying it with a resorbable suture and cutting off the fibroid end.

Once the surgeon has removed all the fibroids he or she judges necessary, the empty capsules are stitched closed with resorbable sutures that slowly dissolve over the following few weeks. If the ligaments supporting the uterus are stretched due to the sheer bulk of the fibroid uterus, these may be tightened by stitching in the equivalent of a small tuck.

Tissues removed during the operation are sent for histology to rule out the possibility of cancerous change in a fibroid (see page 134).

Possible postoperative complications of myomectomy include:

- haemorrhage into the pelvic cavity
- haematoma (filling of capsule spaces with blood and extensive bruising of the uterus)
- uterine scarring
- adhesions (see page 98)
- infection
- uterine rupture during a future pregnancy

It is also not beyond the realms of possibility that endometriosis may be triggered by this surgical invasion of the womb (see page 20).

Unfortunately, myomectomy is not a definitive cure for fibroids. Tiny seedlings are left behind which frequently grow. Studies suggest that up to 45 per cent of women suffer recurrences which may necessitate further surgery.

Of the women who are subfertile and have fibroids, up to 50 per cent conceive following myomectomy. The operation also reduces the risk of miscarriage.

All surgery has an associated risk. The risk of myomectomy seems to be similar to that of hysterectomy, with a small risk of mortality – less than 1 per cent – from complications.

Laser myomectomy at laparotomy

A laser beam can be used rather like a scalpel to cut away fibroids during an open operation. This procedure reduces the amount of blood lost during operation (because the laser seals tissues with heat), reduces tissue inflammation and seems to reduce the amount of post-operative pain.

Although the laser beam can be used to vaporise tissues and destroy fibroids, this is not usually done as tissue samples are needed for examination under the microscope (to rule out cancerous changes).

Laser myomectomy at laparoscopy

Some surgeons have perfected a laparoscopic myomectomy. This technique is not yet widely available but will become so in the near future. The procedure is not suitable for removing multiple fibroids, and most surgeons prefer to use it for removing four or fewer fibroids of small to medium size.

Laparoscopy is undertaken as described on page 53. a laser beam is used like a scalpel to pare away fibroids or shell them out of their capsule. Tissue lumps are cut into smaller pieces inside you and removed through one of the abdominal incisions.

Sometimes a plastic laparoscopy bag is inserted inside you through one of the abdominal incisions and used temporarily to store excised tissue temporarily; the bag is removed at the end of the operation.

Occasionally, large fibroids may be taken out whole through an incision made at the top of the vagina (colpotomy). The fibroid capsule and any incisions are then stitched up using resorbable sutures. (For more information on lasers, see page 90.)

Myolysis

Also called laser drilling, myolysis is a new technique. Six to eight weeks before a myomectomy is to be performed, holes are drilled into deeply embedded intramural, subserosal or submucous fibroids using a laser. This is performed through a laparoscope or hysteroscope, depending on the site of the tumour. The technique reduces fibroid bulk and sets up an inflammatory reaction. As a result, the fibroid separates slightly from its capsule, bulges outwards and becomes less deeply embedded in the uterine wall. Subsequent myomectomy (either by laparotomy or laparoscopy) a few weeks later is then easier and safer, with less cutting required and less risk of haemorrhage.

20

HYSTERECTOMY

A hysterectomy is one of the most emotive operations a woman can have. The word 'hysterectomy' comes from the Greek:

- *hystera* means 'womb'
- *-ectomy* means removal of.

Hysterectomy therefore means removal of the womb.

· *How common is hysterectomy?* ·

Approximately 15 per cent of all women in the UK have had a hysterectomy. It has been estimated that one in five women will have had a hysterectomy or endometrial removal by the age of 55, the commonest reason being for menorrhagia. The introduction of newer, less invasive techniques which remove the endometrium, while keeping the uterine muscular wall intact (endometrial resection or ablation) is likely to make total hysterectomy less common in the future.

Interestingly, women under the age of 30 who have been sterilised are three to four times more likely than average to have a hysterectomy in later life. There are three possible reasons for this:

- Sterilisation may increase the risk of functional uterine disease.
- Surgeons are less reluctant to remove the womb in a woman who has already declared her family complete.
- They stop using the contraceptive pill (which is associated with lighter periods).

The Conditions that can lead to hysterectomy

There are six conditions that, if severe, may result in a woman choosing to have a hysterectomy:

- menorrhagia
- fibroids
- endometriosis
- pelvic inflammatory disease
- prolapse
- cancer.

Hysterectomy is the definitive cure for menorrhagia and fibroids, as neither condition can recur after the operation.

It can greatly relieve the pain of endometriosis and pelvic inflammatory disease, but a more extensive pelvic clearance is needed to give anything approaching a cure.

Whether or not to have a hysterectomy is a decision only you can make, with the guidance of your gynaecologist. Hysterectomy is usually advised if you have:

- not responded to medical treatment of your condition
- heavy bleeding, enough to cause anaemia or to interfere with your lifestyle
- severe pelvic pain – constant or during menstruation – which has not been helped by medication
- a rapidly enlarging uterus with pelvic pressure symptoms, causing problems with urination, defecation or congested circulation (e.g. leading to varicose veins or haemorrhoids)
- completed your family or are aged over 40.

Having made the decision to go ahead, you must next decide whether you should have a vaginal or abdominal operation.

Where possible, hysterectomy is performed vaginally as this is a safer option and avoids an abdominal scar. Until recently, vaginal hysterectomy was not suitable for women who had an immobile uterus or who also needed their ovaries removed. A new technique – laparoscopically assisted vaginal hysterectomy – now enables both the uterus and ovaries to be dissected out and removed via this route. Effectively, most women are now eligible for a vaginal operation, provided their surgeon has the necessary skills.

Some new techniques (ablation, resection) that remove the lining of the womb (to stop or drastically reduce menstrual flow) are now available as surgical alternatives to hysterectomy. These avoid the physical and psychological traumas of a major operation, but are not suitable for treating endometriosis.

If you need an abdominal hysterectomy, there are several options.

· *Total abdominal hysterectomy* ·

Total abdominal hysterectomy (TAH) entails removing your whole uterus, including the cervix. It is usually performed through a bikini-line incision (called a Pfannensteil), but occasionally, where:

- the womb is exceptionally bulky (as with fibroids)
- there is a significant ovarian cyst
- there are widespread adhesions (e.g. from previous pelvic surgery)
- or a malignancy is suspected.

A vertical scar may prove necessary. You will have a catheter

inserted into your bladder to empty it and this may still be in place after
the operation so that you won't have to worry about passing water for a
few days.

The surgeon carefully frees the womb from its supporting ligaments
and blood vessels by clamping off, tying and cutting these structures. If
the ovaries are to remain, the Fallopian tubes are clamped and cut from
the uterus and remain inside too.

An incision is then made around the cervix, into the top end of the
vagina. The freed uterus is then lifted out and sent for examination
under a microscope. The vaginal incision is stitched and the upper
vagina carefully supported so it does not sag downwards. If the ovaries
are left inside, they are usually stitched to the pelvic wall so that they do
not prolapse into the line of fire during sexual intercourse. Any bleeding
points are carefully treated (diathermy or soluble stitches) and the
abdominal wound is then closed. A drain may be left in place for a few
days to suck out any oozing of blood or secretions that collect.

TAH is a major operation, taking several hours. You will need to stop
any hormone treatment (such as the oral contraceptive pill) at least six
weeks beforehand. This is to reduce the risk of post-operative blood
clots while you are immobilised and while the body's clotting state is
increased during the healing process.

You will usually be in hospital for four to seven days after the
operation, although if a complication develops (see page 153) you may
need to stay in for 10–14 days or more.

· *Sub-total hysterectomy* ·

A sub-total hysterectomy was the original type of operation performed.
The womb was dissected out at abdominal operation then sliced off, just
above the cervix, leaving the cervix and vagina intact.

Because the cervix remains, a woman who has this type of
hysterectomy must continue having regular cervical smears, as she is
still at risk of future cervical cancer. This risk is small and will be
minimised by regular cervical screening. In a study of 1,104 Danish
women who underwent sub-total hysterectomy, 2 later developed
cancer of the cervix.

For a while, sub-total hysterectomy went out of fashion and was only
rarely performed. Now, it seems to be making a comeback, especially if
surgery is needed to treat fibroids or menorrhagia. It has the following
possible advantages over the TAH:

- It is an easier operation.
- It reduces the risk of urinary damage during the operation.
- It reduces the risk of future urinary stress incontinence.
- It reduces the risk of future painful intercourse.

- It reduces the risk of bowel problems such as constipation.
- It helps to maintain normal sexual sensations during deep vaginal penetration and orgasm.
- It helps to maintain normal frequency of orgasms.

There is still much controversy over which type of abdominal operation is best. Some surgeons also disagree that a woman's orgasm is affected by the type of operation she has.

· *Wertheim's hysterectomy* ·

This operation is normally performed only when treating cancer but a modified form is occasionally needed to relieve advanced, severe endometriosis. It involves cutting away part of the upper vagina, uterus and cervix, uterine broad ligament, ovaries, Fallopian tubes plus associated lymph glands and fatty tissues if there is a risk of malignant invasion.

· *Vaginal hysterectomy* ·

A vaginal operation has the advantage of no abdominal scar and a quicker post-operative recovery. The vagina can be tightened during the operation, and if you have problems with stress incontinence, the bladder neck can be supported at the same time.

Until recently vaginal hysterectomy was unavailable to women suffering adhesions (bands of internal scar tissue) or those also requiring removal of diseased ovaries. The latest technique, laparo-scopically assisted vaginal hysterectomy, uses a viewing device (laparoscope) and surgical instruments which are inserted through three tiny incisions in the abdominal wall. After gas is inserted to improve access, any adhesions are finely divided under direct visual control and the uterus is quickly and safely excised from its sur-roundings (provided it is no larger than a 12-week pregnancy). The ovaries too, can be excised if necessary.

The abdomen is then deflated and the hysterectomy completed vaginally. Another advantage of this technique is that no internal stitching is involved; an adapted stapling technique is used and women are often able to return home within a few days.

A study in which 42 women were discharged from hospital within three to five days of surgery found that only two needed readmission – one for haemorrhage, and one for constipation. Two others developed a urinary tract infection which was treated by their GP. Six weeks after discharge, 28 out of 30 women discharged on the third day, 3 out of 5 discharged on the fourth and 6 out of 7 discharged on the fifth were more than happy to have been able to convalesce at home.

Vaginal hysterectomy may eventually be performed as an outpatient procedure. A new technique is so simple it has cut operating time down to 15 minutes. The procedure uses a new, automatic stapling device to repair tissues after the womb is removed. Of eight women who underwent the first trial, all were mobile within a few hours of the operation and were able to go home the next day. The procedure is currently undergoing a randomised trial to compare it with the more conventional vaginal hysterectomy.

· *Removal of the ovaries* ·

In younger women, the ovaries are retained where possible to prevent an early menopause. They can safely be left inside if the hysterectomy is performed for fibroids, but some women go on to develop ovarian pain from residual ovary syndrome, or cyclical premenstrual syndrome.

Between 1 and 5 per cent of women whose ovaries are conserved will need surgery in the future to have them removed.

If you have endometriosis, your ovaries must be removed during hysterectomy, otherwise any residual peritoneal endometrial implants will remain active. If ovaries are retained, 13 per cent of women will have a recurrence of endometriosis within three years, and 40 per cent after five years. The more severe the endometriosis, the more likely it is to recur.

Older women having a hysterectomy for fibroids may have their ovaries removed if they look diseased (e.g. cysts, endometriomas) or if the menopause is approaching.

Removal of the ovaries and Fallopian tubes is called a bilateral salpingo-oophorectomy (BSO). You may therefore see your operation booked as a TAH & BSO (total abdominal hysterectomy plus bilateral salpingo-oophorectomy).

The disadvantage of having the ovaries out is that you will have an instant surgically induced menopause. If the operation is for fibroids, you can start hormone replacement therapy (HRT) straight away. If you have endometriosis, you will need to wait at least six months for any remaining lesions to wither away before HRT is started.

Occasionally a small fragment of ovary may remain inside your abdomen after a TAH & BSO. This may be enough to continue cyclical stimulation of your endometrial lesions, so that if your operation was for endometriosis your pain may continue. Although this risk is small, it is worth discussing it with your consultant before the operation.

The advantage of having your ovaries removed – especially as the menopause approaches – is that you will never develop ovarian cancer.

It is estimated that 1 in 500 women whose ovaries are conserved in the population at large will develop an ovarian malignancy.

· *Possible complications of hysterectomy* ·

Although hysterectomy has a low mortality rate (6 per 10,000 abdominal operations – less for vaginal ones) between 25 and 50 per cent of patients suffer a complication. Most of these are minor and easily remedied, but a few are serious. The possible complications of hysterectomy include:

- urinary tract infection
- chest infection
- wound infection
- pelvic abscess
- haemorrhage (during or after the operation)
- damage to other pelvic organs (bladder, bowel,
- ureter, blood vessels, ovaries)
- deep pain during sexual intercourse
- vaginal prolapse
- urinary stress incontinence
- future bowel problems (e.g. constipation)
- blood clots and pulmonary embolism.

· *After the operation* ·

Women are discharged home increasingly early after a hysterectomy, and the GP is entrusted with their post-operative care. In one study (1992) the average hospital stay for TAH was 4.4 days, but only 2.4 days for laparoscopically assisted vaginal hysterectomy. Recovery, too, was quicker with the vaginal than with the abdominal operation. Full recovery generally takes:

- 6–8 weeks for TAH
- 5 weeks for vaginal hysterectomy
- 3 weeks for laparoscopic hysterectomy.

Return to work may take longer, while emotional recovery and coming to terms with no longer being fertile may take a year or more. Every woman differs, and no one can guarantee how quickly you will get over what is essentially a major physical and psychological operation.

Lifting heavy objects and strenuous exercise are usually discouraged for six weeks following hysterectomy to allow internal healing to take place. When you can return to driving a car depends on your insurance company; some will not provide cover for six weeks post-operatively, so be sure to check this.

· *Hysterectomy and your sex life* ·

Generally, a woman who has had a hysterectomy can resume sexual relations as soon as any discharge and tenderness have settled down.

Some doctors suggest waiting until after the six-week clinic check, and in practice most women avoid penetrative sex for several weeks from a desire to allow everything to heal up. When resuming sex, follow these simple rules:

- Take your time during sex
- Use water-based gels or pessaries for lubrication
- Experiment to find which position is most comfortable
- If anything hurts – stop!

Psychological problems, such as depression, feelings of lost femininity and lowered sex drive, may occur after hysterectomy. Proper counselling before and after the operation is essential. If a woman reaches her own decision about the necessity of a hysterectomy, fewer emotional problems tend to occur. Often, a woman is so grateful for the cessation of pain, menorrhagia or premenstrual syndrome that the operation transforms her life – especially her sex drive.

If your ovaries are removed, sudden withdrawal of oestrogen can lead to post-operative depression, lowered sex drive and vaginal dryness as part of early menopausal symptoms. If HRT is prescribed six weeks after the operation, your symptoms will improve (see page 160).

Many women find that their orgasm feels different after the hysterectomy. A study in Japan found that 27 per cent of hysterectomised women experienced loss of uterine sensation while making love and 70 per cent claimed difficulty in reaching an orgasm.

A similar survey in Finland compared women who had had a total abdominal hysterectomy with those who'd had a sub-total hysterectomy in which the cervix was left intact. Researchers found no difference in sexual desire between the two groups, but after one year the women who had a sub-total operation enjoyed a significantly higher frequency of orgasms than women who had undergone a total hysterectomy.

During orgasm, deep muscular contractions occur. These involve the uterus and attached ligaments and some of these sensations will disappear after hysterectomy. Some women find this enhances and intensifies their clitoral sensations and claim their enjoyment of orgasm is improved – especially if their sex life was virtually nonexistent before due to pelvic congestion or constant pelvic pain.

21

ENDOMETRIAL ABLATION AS AN ALTERNATIVE TO HYSTERECTOMY

Lasers, hot cutting wires and microwaves are rapidly taking over from the traditional surgeon's knife. At least 50 per cent of women undergoing hysterectomy are eligible for the alternative of destruction or removal of just the endometrium, via the vagina and cervix. This leaves the wall of the uterus intact and is a safer, less invasive alternative to hysterectomy. These options are not suitable for women who have endometriosis, adenomyosis or large fibroids, for although they will solve the problem of heavy, painful bleeding, they will not affect ectopic endometrial lesions or symptoms due to fibroid bulk.

The aim of these new techniques is to remove the entire thickness of the endometrium so the operation should result in cessation of periods. Often, however, small strips of endometrial tissue are left behind, resulting in light monthly bleeds.

Like hysterectomy, the procedure should be performed only in women who do not want further pregnancies, as most of those who have it are rendered sterile.

Drugs are usually prescribed to thin the endometrium down prior to resection or ablation. These include danazol and GnRH analogues.

Various techniques are available for removing the endometrium. These include:

- resection
- laser ablation
- rollerball diathermy
- radiofrequency
- thermal (microwave) ablation
- cryo (freezing) ablation.

Only the first two techniques are in frequent use. A survey in 1990 showed that over 60 per cent of gynaecological surgical units offered endometrial ablation. Of these, 77 per cent were using endometrial resection, while 22 per cent used laser ablation.

Radiofrequency endometrial ablation heats the endometrium with radiofrequency electromagnetic energy through a probe inserted via the cervix. In 1991, only two UK units used the procedure, and at least one of these has now abandoned the technique.

Rollerball ablation is popular in the US, where it is used more frequently than resection. The electro-coagulation technique is still uncommon in the UK.

The different procedures seem to have similar success rates. Studies suggest that 20–40 per cent of women have complete amenorrhoea (no periods), while 40–60 per cent have a significantly reduced menstrual flow. After rollerball ablation, 30 per cent of women stopped having periods, 27 per cent had slight staining or spotting each month and 28 per cent continued having light periods. Surprisingly, 7 per cent of women claimed to notice no change in their periods, while 8 per cent continued experiencing what they would describe as a normal menstrual flow (that is, reduced from their previous menorrhagia).

Some women need to undergo a repeat resection. These failures may be partly due to the learning curve each surgeon must go through while gaining experience in a new hysteroscopic technique.

After any procedure to remove the endometrium, a woman will have a persistent blood-stained watery discharge for several months. This is normal. As a result, the effectiveness of the resection/ablation may not become obvious until four to six months after surgery was performed.

Hysteroscopic endometrial transcervical resection

The endometrium is first thinned down by a course of danazol or GnRH analogue. A general anaesthetic or epidural is used. A viewing instrument with an attached hot cutting loop (resectoscope) is then inserted into the uterus. The loop electro-cuts and cauterises endometrial tissues, paring away the endometrium down as far as the underlying uterine muscle.

The advantage of this procedure over laser ablation is that parings can be collected and sent for examination under a microscope to rule out a missed endometrial carcinoma (rare).

There is a 2 per cent risk of uterine perforation with this technique. Provided there are no complications, you can expect to go home the same day and return to work within two weeks.

In one study, 90 per cent of women enjoyed a significant improvement in symptoms throughout the follow-up period of two-and-a-half years. Menstruation ceased in 42 per cent of cases; 4 per cent of the women needed a subsequent hysterectomy due to failure of the procedure.

Hysteroscopic endometrial laser ablation

In this procedure the endometrium is initially thinned down by a course of danazol or GnRH analogue drugs. You are given a general anaesthetic (or an epidural) and a neodymium-YAG laser fitted to a hysteroscope is inserted into the uterus. Saline is continuously flushed into the uterus to distend the uterine cavity, flush away vaporised tissue and provide a clear view. Under direct visual control, the laser beam is then systematically dragged over the endometrial surface. Tissues are vaporised down as far as the underlying uterine muscle. The disadvantage of this procedure is that no tissue parings are available for examination under the microscope. Endometrial biopsy to rule out endometrial carcinoma is therefore often carried out before the procedure starts.

You can expect to go home the same day and probably return to work within two weeks.

In one study, of 479 women followed up for at least six months following one or two laser ablations, 97 per cent had a satisfactory response but 3 per cent required a subsequent hysterectomy. A complete cessation of periods was achieved in 60 per cent, while 32 per cent had a satisfactory reduction in menstrual flow. Of 8 per cent who failed to improve after the first ablation, two-thirds were happy after the procedure was repeated. (For more information about lasers, see page 90.)

Combined resection ablation

Some surgeons have perfected the use of endometrial resection and laser ablation together, using a resectoscope that has a laser channel. This speeds the resection up, and reduces the risk of perforation as the laser is used in the thinner areas of the uterus (fundus and horns).

Endometrial microwave ablation

A new technique using microwaves to destroy the endometrium is currently undergoing trials. The intra-uterine probe consists of an angled metal rod. This is inserted into the vagina and rotated around 360 degrees to reach the two corners, or horns, of the womb. The probe generates a heat gradient across the endometrium which effectively kills endometrial cells at a temperature of 53–63°C. Uterine muscle is heated to only 38–40° C (similar to a high fever) and escapes unharmed.

The popularity of these hysteroscopic procedures

Interestingly, research suggests that women with heavy periods are more likely to be satisfied after a hysterectomy than with minimally invasive hysteroscopic techniques, despite their faster recovery time, reduced risk of complications and decreased pain. Studies show that all women undergoing hysterectomy need painkillers, compared with only 16 per cent of women having endometrial resection.

It is the finality of hysterectomy that makes many women prefer it. In one study, 204 women were randomly assigned to either traditional hysterectomy or endometrial resection/ablation. After a year, 89 per cent of women who had had a hysterectomy were 'very satisfied' with the outcome, having taken two to three months to recover. In comparison, only 78 per cent of patients in the other group were 'very satisfied' despite having taken only two to four weeks to recover. This was probably because in this trial, resection/ablation provided only an average 50 per cent reduction in menstrual flow.

Women who continue to have cyclical menstrual bleeding after endometrial resection/ablation may need to continue using an effective method of contraception. Ask your doctor for advice.

Women who are not eligible for these procedures

Women who are not eligible for these procedures include those who have a malignancy of the reproductive tract and those whose conditions (e.g. large fibroids, endometriosis, pelvic adhesions) would not be expected to improve through removal of the endometrium alone.

Possible complications of hysteroscopic procedures

- haemorrhage
- uterine perforation with damage to other pelvic organs (e.g. bladder, ureter, bowel, major blood vessels); this is more common with resection than laser ablation
- temporary fluid overload from absorption of the saline used to hold the walls of the uterus apart during hysteroscopy
- collection of blood in the womb (haematometra)
- infection of the endometrium
- urinary tract infection
- chest infection (if general anaesthetic used)
- post-operative blood clotting disorders
- increased painful periods afterwards
- intrauterine adhesions (synechiae).

22

THE MENOPAUSE AND HRT

Both endometriosis and fibroids are oestrogen-dependent and naturally shrink when oestrogen levels fall at the menopause. Occasionally, oestrogen levels remain high enough after the menopause to maintain these diseases, usually where oestrogen continues to be secreted by fatty tissues, in obese women, or where HRT is prescribed.

The menopause is defined as the time when the last period occurs. This can be diagnosed only in retrospect after a woman of suitable age, with classic symptoms, has not had a period for one year.

The menopause is triggered by the ovaries running out of eggs. A five-month-old female fetus contains around 7 million eggs. By the time of birth, this number falls to 2 million and by the time of puberty less than half a million remain. The rest have slowly degenerated and resorbed in a process known as atresia. No new eggs are ever formed after birth. During each monthly cycle, an average of 15 eggs start to mature and are then abandoned as a single dominant follicle takes over (see page 8). Many eggs continue the slow process of attrition, so that by the age of 50, few if any eggs remain.

As fewer and fewer eggs develop in each menstrual cycle, the level of oestrogen falls. The pituitary gland senses this and tries to kick-start the tiring ovaries by increasing its secretion of follicle stimulating hormone (FSH – see page 7).

The dwindling number of eggs mature irregularly, so that as the menopause approaches, the length of your menstrual cycles varies and periods become irregular.

Menstruation stops when the ovaries literally run out of eggs. As oestrogen levels fall, the endometrium loses its main source of stimulation and periods stop altogether. Your last actual period denotes the date of the menopause itself.

For most women, the last natural period will occur between the ages of 45 and 55, with an average in the UK of 51 (49 in the USA) years. Interestingly, when a woman has a hysterectomy with her ovaries left in place, 25 per cent of women experience menopausal symptoms within two years of operation. Overall, the average age of the menopause for hysterectomised women (whose ovaries are left intact) is four years earlier than normal at 47 (45 in the USA) years. The reason remains unknown, but the most likely explanation is that the operation has an adverse effect on ovarian blood supply. An alternative theory is that an as-yet unrecognised interaction occurs between the ovaries and the uterus, such that early ovarian failure is triggered by hysterectomy.

Another major factor influencing the age a woman experiences menopause is smoking. The more you smoke, the sooner your periods cease; heavy smokers tend to reach the menopause two years earlier than non-smokers.

· *Symptoms* ·

Many of the symptoms of the menopause are related to withdrawal of oestrogen and to the side effects of increasing FSH levels. These symptoms include:

- hot flushes
- night sweats
- vaginal dryness
- loss of sex drive
- difficulties with intercourse
- urinary symptoms
- skin dryness and ageing.

Hot flushes are the commonest symptom, experienced by at least 80 per cent of menopausal women. Other symptoms include irritability, depression, aches, pains and tiredness.

· *Hormone replacement therapy* ·

Hormone replacement therapy (HRT) is designed to give back some of the hormones your ovaries have stopped making. It consists of a natural form of the female hormone oestrogen, plus (if the woman still has an intact uterus) a synthetic progestogen. Progesterone is essential to protect the endometrium from over-stimulation which is linked with an increased risk of cancer. Progesterone is given for 10–14 days, then stopped to trigger endometrial shedding. This mimics a period, but is more correctly known as a withdrawal bleed.

HRT may be prescribed:

- following a natural menopause, after your periods have stopped
- after surgical removal of the uterus and ovaries
- to counteract menopausal symptoms during the early menopause before your periods have stopped
- as an add-back protective treatment when a chemical menopause is induced by some drugs (see page 84).

· *HRT preparations* ·

Oestrogen taken by mouth is absorbed from the stomach and is partially broken down in the liver before reaching its target sites such as the skin, breasts and vagina. Oral preparations of HRT therefore contain higher doses than HRT delivered via another route such as a subcutaneous implant (under the skin) or a skin patch. Implants are inserted under local anaesthetic and last for up to six months before needing replacement. Skin patches are stuck onto the skin of the lower abdomen and replaced twice a week. If you have an intact uterus, you will need to take progesterone for some days of your cycle as well.

Oestrogen can also be given as a cream to reduce vaginal dryness and tissue shrinkage.

A new preparation, an oestrogen gel rubs onto the skin is now available in the UK. It has been used with great success in France for over 20 years, where it is the most popular form of HRT.

· *HRT and menstruation* ·

If you have an intact uterus, most HRT causes a monthly withdrawal bleed as part of the way it protects the endometrium from over-stimulation and pre-cancerous changes. This return or continuation of periods is a major reason why many women give up treatment or decide not to start it in the first place.

One synthetic hormone, tibolone, has both oestrogen and progesterone effects. It can therefore control oestrogen withdrawal symptoms without the need for a withdrawal bleed. It works best in women who have not had a period for at least one year.

Another way of taking HRT continuously without a regular pill-free break (and with no risky return of periods) has also just been introduced.

· *The risks and benefits of HRT* ·

It is important to realise that the oestrogens used in HRT are very different from those used in the combined oral contraceptive pill.

In women experiencing ovarian failure, HRT restores oestrogen levels to the low normal range. The total monthly dose taken is much less than would be secreted by the ovaries in a normal menstrual cycle. The contraceptive pill, on the other hand, deliberately increases hormone levels above normal to approximate those of pregnancy. These high doses artificially suppress ovarian activity.

Also, the type of oestrogen used in the contraceptive pill is usually synthetic whereas HRT tends to contain natural oestrogens. For both the above reasons, the risks and benefits of HRT are different from those of the Pill.

The side effects of HRT are usually minor. They tend to occur at the start of treatment and to settle down within a few weeks. Mild reactions are sometimes helped by changing the dosage or type of HRT. Some, however, are troublesome enough for treatment to be stopped.

HRT and coronary heart disease

Studies show that HRT reduces the risk of coronary heart disease in women past the menopause by up to 50 per cent. In women who have already had a heart attack, HRT provides 80 per cent protection against another one occurring. As a 50-year-old woman not on HRT has a 46 per cent chance of developing coronary heart disease and a 31 per cent chance of dying from it, the protection from HRT is significant.

Oestrogen has this effect by lowering harmful blood cholesterol levels (LDLs), by preserving arterial wall elasticity and by discouraging atherosclerosis (hardening and furring up of the arteries).

HRT and osteoporosis

HRT provides significant protection against osteoporosis. A 50-year-old woman has an overall 50 per cent chance of sustaining an osteoporotic bone fracture during the rest of her life and a 3 per cent chance of dying as a result. The specific injuries include:

- a 15 per cent risk of hip fracture
- a 16 per cent risk of wrist fracture
- a 20–30 per cent risk of spinal deformity from vertebral collapse.

Oestrogen has a beneficial effect on bone cells to reduce bone resorption and to increase bone laying down. As a result, HRT reduces the risk of a hip fracture by up to 40 per cent. Bone loss resumes once oestrogen therapy stops, and unfortunately studies indicate that protection against osteoporosis is lost within five years of coming off HRT.

HRT and breast cancer

One worrying association with HRT is the risk of developing breast cancer. A 50-year-old woman not on HRT has an 10 per cent risk of developing breast cancer during the rest of her life and a 3 per cent chance of dying from it.

Studies suggest that using HRT for more than eight years increases this risk of breast cancer by 25 per cent over ten years, giving an overall risk of 12.5 per cent as opposed to the normal risk of 10 per cent. The risk seems to be greatest in those who have a history of benign breast problems, or who have a mother, sister or daughter with breast cancer.

However, it does not seem to increase the risk of dying from breast cancer. Women using HRT before developing breast cancer may actually have a lower risk of death from breast cancer than those not taking HRT, because stopping HRT causes an oestrogen-dependent tumour to shrink.

The best medical advice at present is that using HRT for five to eight years will provide maximum benefit against heart disease and minimum risk of breast cancer.

Overall risk assessment of HRT

Taking all risks and benefits of HRT into account, the life expectancy of a 50-year-old woman taking combined oestrogen-progestogen HRT is expected to rise by almost a year according to computer simulations. However, women who already have an increased risk of breast cancer (that is one or two first-degree relatives with the disease) gain little or no increased life expectancy from HRT.

Taking HRT for five years minimises the risk of developing breast cancer and strongly protects against heart attack. It also buys the skeleton five crucial years against osteoporosis and improves quality of life by controlling menopausal symptoms.

Decisions about taking HRT involve individual subjective judgments. Some women regard the small increased risk of breast cancer as more important than the large reduction in risk of heart disease – especially if

---

SIDE EFFECTS OF HRT

- gastrointestinal upsets
- nausea and vomiting
- weight gain
- breast tenderness and enlargement
- breakthrough bleeding
- headaches or migraine
- dizziness
- leg cramps
- increase in size of uterine fibroids
- intolerance of contact lenses
- skin reactions
- loss of scalp hair or increased body or facial hair – these changes are due to the different hormone sensitivities of hair follicles in different parts of the body
- premenstrual syndrome.

HRT SHOULD NOT BE TAKEN BY WOMEN WHO:

- are pregnant or breast-feeding
- have had an oestrogen-dependent cancer (e.g. of the breast) unless their doctor agrees. Some experts feel that women who have been successfully treated for cancer and have no evidence of a recurrence can sometimes take HRT
- have undiagnosed vaginal bleeding
- have active endometriosis
- have active blood clotting disorders
- have severe heart, liver or kidney disease.

HRT SHOULD BE USED ONLY WITH CAUTION IN WOMEN WHO HAVE:

- migraines
- gallstones
- a history of blood clotting disorders
- mild ongoing liver disease
- a type of deafness called otosclerosis
- had skin itching during pregnancy (pruritis)
- a rare blistering skin disease of pregnancy called pemphigoid gestationis
- multiple sclerosis
- epilepsy
- diabetes
- high blood pressure
- a rare metabolic disease called porphyria
- fibroids of the womb
- a nervous and muscular condition called tetany.

---

a friend or relative has suffered from breast cancer. Other women may want, above all, to prevent hip fracture or osteoporotic wedge fractures of the vertebrae resulting in spinal deformity.

The severity of menopausal symptoms is certainly controlled by using HRT and some women opt to take HRT for six to twelve months to see them through this difficult period.

For women who are unable to take HRT, menopausal flushes can be helped by a prescribed drug called clonidine.

Otherwise, symptoms can be helped naturally by following the dietary, exercise and relaxation advice in Chapter 23.

23

SELF HELP: ENDOMETRIOSIS, FIBROIDS AND THE MENOPAUSE

There are many things you can do yourself to help to ease symptoms caused by endometriosis, fibroids or the menopause. These include paying attention to your diet, taking regular exercise and using relaxation techniques to reduce tension.

· *Diet* ·

Some edible plants seem to have a beneficial influence on human hormone status. These include:

- soya products (such as soybeans, soymeal, tofu)
- fibre-rich unrefined grain products (such as rye)
- nuts and seeds
- beans
- pulses
- peas
- berries
- dried fruits
- cruciferous plants – members of the cabbage and turnip family – especially the more exotic varieties such as kohlrabi and Chinese leaves.

These plants are a rich source of isoflavonoids – weak plant oestrogens that are converted into biologically active hormone-like substances in your gut by the fermentation reactions of intestinal bacteria. These plant oestrogens are then reabsorbed to have a beneficial effect on health. Paradoxically, rather than encouraging hormone-related diseases such as breast cancer, prostate cancer, endometriosis and fibroids, they may help to protect against them by inhibiting the body's own oestrogens.

Plant oestrogens seem to reduce exposure to the body's own oestrogens by increasing production of sex hormone binding globulin (SHBG) – a carrier protein that mops up natural oestrogens and binds them so they are not available to act on hormone-responsive tissues such as tumours, endometrial implants and fibroids. Isoflavonoid phytoestrogens also seem to have a direct effect on human hormone production and metabolism plus a damping-down effect on tumour cell growth.

Fibre

People following a low-fibre diet have higher oestrogen levels than those on a healthier, high-fibre diet. Oestrogens are quickly extracted from the circulation by your liver, chemically altered and excreted out through the bile into the intestines. Some oestrogens are reabsorbed from the gut to go round your system again. This is called the enterohepatic circulation. Oestrogen levels can vary enormously at any particular time in the menstrual cycle, depending on how much oestrogen is reabsorbed. Following a high-fibre diet seems to bind excreted oestrogen in the bowel and reduce the amount that is reabsorbed.

This suggests that following a high-fibre diet will reduce your exposure to natural (endogenous) oestrogens and reduce their effects on conditions such as endometriosis and fibroids.

Dietary antioxidants

Yellow, orange, red and green vegetables and fruits are rich in the protective antioxidant vitamins C, E and betacarotene. These help to reduce cell damage (which might trigger tumours such as fibroids and gynaecological cancers) by neutralising damaging chemicals produced as offshoots of your metabolic reactions. These highly reactive chemicals are called free radicals.

As its name suggests, a free radical is a highly unstable entity that races round picking fights and causing damage. The molecular version carries a negative charge which it desperately tries to unload. Each body cell is bombarded with an estimated 100,000 oxidating reactions every day; the number is twice as high in smokers.

If molecular DNA is damaged through these oxidations, errors can occur when your genetic material is copied during cell division. It is possible that these errors can trigger cancers or benign tumours such as fibroids. Following a diet rich in vitamins C, E and betacarotene may help to prevent these.

The American National Cancer Institute recommends a daily intake of at least 6mg of betacarotene to decrease the risk of cancer. Most of us get less than 2mg per day from our diet.

Some experts suggest taking high doses of some vitamin supplements for their antioxidant effects:

- 15mg betacarotene
- 150–300mg vitamin C
- 30–40mg vitamin E.

If you don't want to take supplements, make sure your diet contains foods rich in these micronutrients.

Foods rich in vitamin C include:
- blackcurrants
- guavas
- kiwi fruit
- citrus fruit
- mangoes
- green peppers
- strawberries
- green sprouting vegetables such as broccoli, sprouts, watercress, parsley
- potatoes.

Foods rich in vitamin E include:
- wheatgerm oil
- avocado pear
- margarine
- eggs
- butter
- wholemeal cereals
- seeds
- nuts
- bread
- oily fish
- broccoli.

Foods rich in betacarotene include:
- dark green leafy vegetables and yellow-orange fruits
- carrots
- sweet potatoes
- spinach
- broccoli
- parsley
- watercress
- spring greens
- cantaloupe melons
- apricots
- peaches
- mangoes
- red and yellow peppers
- tomatoes
- sweet corn.

Dietary saturated fat

New research shows that people who eat a typical Western diet high in animal (saturated) fat and low in fruit, vegetables and fibre have an increased risk of certain hormone-related cancers.

Red meat is the food with the strongest positive link to advanced hormonal diseases such as endometrial cancer. In one study, women who ate large quantities of meat and fatty foods were found to be up to four times at risk of contracting endometrial cancer compared with women who ate little red meat and concentrated on a diet high in fruit, vegetables and fibre. Butter trebled the risk at highest intakes; sugar, eggs, ham and beef doubled the risk at highest intakes.

Eating a vegetarian diet of macrobiotic vegetables, wholegrains, bread and pasta appears to cut the risk of endometrial cancer by about 60 per cent, while eating at least 2–3 pieces of fresh fruit per day halves the risk.

· *Exercise* ·

Regular exercise has many health benefits. Exercise needs to be brisk enough to work up a light sweat and to raise your pulse to between 120 and 130 beats per minute (unless you have a heart problem – consult your doctor). Ideally, you need to exercise every day for at least 20 minutes, or three times per week for 30 minutes each session.

Interestingly, regular exercise has been shown to eliminate many of the unwanted side effects of danazol (see page 78).

This may be because exercise increases the number of male hormone receptors (androceptors) in muscles, which limits the androgenic (masculinising) side effects of the drug. It also helps to prevent weight gain and to increase feelings of wellbeing.

Regular exercise has also been shown to reduce the incidence of:

- menopausal symptoms
- fatigue
- low mood swings
- obesity
- respiratory problems
- coronary heart disease
- diabetes
- osteoporosis
- high blood pressure
- stroke
- constipation
- uterine cancer
- colorectal cancer.

Pelvic exercises

Many women with endometriosis and fibroids suffer from symptoms of pelvic congestion, especially in the premenstrual phase of the monthly cycle.

This congestion can be relieved to a certain extent by pelvic exercises. These tone up pelvic floor muscle, stimulate pelvic circulation and help to drain away excess fluid. Although pelvic exercises have not been scientifically proven to relieve pelvic congestion, there is anecdotal evidence to suggest that it can relieve premenstrual feelings of congestion and even encourage fibroids to shrink.

So-called pelvic sitz baths are recommended to stimulate pelvic circulation. These involve sitting alternately in a bidet/bath of cold water for three minutes, then hot water for three minutes, alternating the two at least three times.

Then practise pelvic rocking exercises for five minutes while standing up. Move your pelvis to and fro, repeatedly squeezing your buttocks together and tightening your pelvic floor muscles. The easiest way to identify these is to practise trying to stop the flow of urine midstream when you next open your bladder. The muscles you need to tighten to do this are the muscles you need to clench repeatedly (along with your buttocks) during your pelvic rocking exercise.

· *Healthy diet and lifestyle tips* ·

The following advice may help to ease symptoms of fibroids and endometriosis. They may also reduce the risk of gynaecological cancers.

- Lose excess weight (adipose tissue synthesises oestrogens).
- If you smoke, try to cut down gradually.
- Restrict alcohol intake – preferably to a maximum of three or four alcoholic drinks per week.

Reduce your dietary intake of:

- sugar and sweetened foods
- artificial sweeteners
- white-flour products
- fast food and junk food
- salt
- red meat – limit yourself to one or two portions per week (preferably less)
- tea, coffee and fizzy drinks
- fatty foods, especially saturated dairy products

Try to limit your fat intake to a total of 25 per cent of daily calories (fat counters, available in newsagents, can help you do this). It is suggested that restricting fat intake to 10 per cent would prevent up to 35 per cent of all tumours, but this diet is difficult to follow.

Increase your dietary intake of:

- fish, especially oily fish (salmon, herring, sardines, mackerel); if possible take it Japanese style, ultra fresh and raw (as in sushi, sashimi)
- fresh vegetables and fruit; the World Health Organisation (WHO) recommend a minimum of five portions fresh fruit, vegetables or saladstuff per day, to a weight of around 400g (five portions per day; organic if possible)
- phytoestrogen-rich foods such as soy, cruciferous plants, rye
- unrefined carbohydrates such as wholemeal bread, brown rice, wholewheat pasta, wholegrains, to WHO recommendations of 50–70 per cent of energy intake
- fibre – at least 30–40g per day
- nuts; for their essential fatty acid content – they help to even out hormonal imbalances that are linked with cyclical breast pain, eczema and premenstrual syndrome
- cold-pressed vegetable oils (such as olive, sunflower, safflower, linseed) in place of animal fats
- low-fat versions of dairy products; try to drink up to 600ml of skimmed or semi-skimmed milk per day
- mineral water – try to drink three to six large glasses of water daily, preferably filtered or bottled.

· *Supplements* ·

Many people have reduced intakes of essential vitamins and minerals. The government-funded Dietary and Nutritional Survey of British Adults (1990) found that the average British female obtained less than the new EC recommended daily intakes of the following:

- vitamin A
- betacarotene
- thiamin
- vitamin B6
- biotin
- pantothenic acid
- vitamin C

- vitamin D
- vitamin E
- iron
- calcium
- magnesium
- zinc

Even when average intakes seemed adequate, it must be remembered that an average is only an average. 50 per cent of people obtain less than the mean average figure.

Everyone, but especially those with symptoms of a body malfunction, should take a careful look at their diet to ensure they are getting enough basic micronutrients. The Endometriosis Society suggests that increasing your intake of certain nutrients can help to ease some endometriosis symptoms.

If you are unable to adjust your diet, it is worth trying a course of a good vitamin and mineral supplement for a few months to see if it improves your symptoms.

Higher intakes of vitamins C, E and betacarotene than the recommended minimums are suggested for their antioxidant actions.

Supplements and your drugs

Some women have found that taking evening primrose oil helps to reduce some of the side effects of danazol, such as tiredness, depression, mood swings and water retention, at a dose of 2–3x500mg capsules twice daily. Linseed oil, too, is rich in the beneficial oils found in evening primrose oil.

Other women have found that vitamin B6 (pyridoxine) helps to reduce their danazol side effects. This is best taken as part of a vitamin B complex for a balanced intake. Vitamin B6 is essential for the proper functioning of more than 60 enzymes and for regulating the function of sex hormones.

You need around 2mg of vitamin B6 per day. Research suggests that some people need slightly more – but only up to 5–10mg per day. Do not take doses of vitamin B6 higher than 50mg per day for longer than a month. After a month, drop back to a daily intake of 5–10mg per day unless advised differently by your doctor (because you have a proven vitamin B6 deficiency). This is because regular intake of excessive vitamin B6 can produce symptoms of nerve damage.

Symptoms due to too much vitamin B6:
- tingling
- burning
- shooting pains
- pins and needles (paraesthesiae)
- clumsiness
- unsteadiness on the feet
- numbness
- depression
- headache
- tiredness.

Many women with gynaecological problems take large doses of vitamin B6. This may in fact make their symptoms worse. In extreme cases, when massive doses of 500mg per day or more are used, excess vitamin B6 can lead to partial paralysis.

Foods rich in vitamin B6 include:
- yeast extract
- whole-grain cereals
- liver
- soya flour
- bananas
- walnuts
- meat
- oily fish
- brown rice
- green, leafy vegetables
- avocado
- egg yolk
- royal jelly.

Vitamin B6 is destroyed by cooking and by exposure to light – so wholefood diets containing raw foods will be richest in this important nutrient.

Complementary therapies and endometriosis

Complementary therapies are designed to be used alongside traditional medical and surgical treatments for a variety of problems. You may find that one of the following therapies helps you.

Acupuncture is based on the belief that life energy (Chi or Qi) flows through the body along channels known as meridians. By inserting fine needles into acupuncture points overlying these meridians, the practitioner can, it is believed, overcome blockages and correct or alter the flow of Chi to relieve symptoms. The best-known effect of Chi manipulation is local anaesthesia. Research suggests that acupuncture causes the release of natural, heroin-like chemicals that act as painkillers. Acupuncture can help most conditions including stress, heavy painful periods, menopausal symptoms, premenstrual syndrome, pelvic pain and sexual problems.

Acupressure is similar to acupuncture, but instead of inserting needles at points along the meridian, the practitioner stimulates the points using firm thumb pressure or fingertip massage. The best-known example of acupressure is Shiatsu (see below).

The Alexander Technique is based on the belief that poor posture and faulty body movements contribute to disease. By teaching people to stand and move correctly, without undue stress, the Alexander Technique aims to improve ill health. The principles are used to treat a wide variety of conditions, including asthma, rheumatism, back pain, stuttering, stress and depression.

Aromatherapy uses a variety of techniques (e.g. inhalation, massage, bathing) to administer aromatic, essential oils extracted from plants. These are particularly effective in treating stress or emotional problems. The intense aroma of essential oils stimulates the olfactory nerves running from the nose to the limbic system of the brain, where emotional responses are centred. Oils may also be absorbed through the skin to have a therapeutic effect. Too much can be harmful, however, and it is important that oils be chosen with care and used according to instruction.

Bach Flower Remedies are homoeopathic remedies prepared from flower essences and brandy. There are 38 different flower remedies used to treat a variety of emotional symptoms. Bach Rescue Remedy is an excellent homoeopathic treatment for stress, pain and life's ups and downs.

Flotation therapy is a relaxation technique in which you float on top of a solution of salt water more buoyant than the Dead Sea. Light, sound, temperature and the effects of gravity are removed to produce profound relaxation. Theta brain waves are induced which produce buzzes of creative thought. Flotation can reduce high blood pressure, lower cholesterol levels, relieve chronic pain and reduce the effects of stress.

Healing uses the powers of faith, spiritualism or psychic energy to improve physical or emotional symptoms. Powers are often channelled through the hands, although some therapists project healing over long distances. Those being treated often feel sensations of heat, cold or tingling on the skin, but no known form of transmitted energy has yet been identified.

Herbal medicine is widely practised by Chinese and Indian doctors. Patients are prescribed individual blends of herbs on the basis of symptoms, signs, diet and lifestyle. Prescriptions are then changed as symptoms change. Herbalism can help most kinds of illness, even long-standing conditions, such as endometriosis, arthritis, migraine and eczema, where orthodox medicine sometimes fails. Some herbal medicines need to be brewed to make a decoction for drinking.

Homoeopathy is based on the two principles: 'like cures like' and 'less cures more.' It uses natural substances that, if used full-strength, would produce symptoms in a healthy person similar to those of the illness it is designed to treat. By diluting these substances many millions of times, homeopathy enhances their curative properties while removing their underdesirable side effects. Homoeopathic remedies aim to stimulate the body's natural healing forces to produce relief. They can also help you to recover from the effects of medical or surgical treatment. A new homoeopathic treatment (Endobrit) is currently undergoing trials to treat endometriosis and is looking promising. It should be available in the UK soon.

Hypnotherapy uses the powerful tools of suggestion and relaxation to relieve anxiety and stress. Conditions such as eczema, migraine, peptic ulcers, irritable bowel syndrome, asthma and insomnia are often improved.

Massage is one of the oldest complementary therapies known. It is particularly useful in helping tension, circulatory problems, high blood pressure, insomnia, depression, back pain and muscular aches. There are many different types of massage, using a variety of rubbing, drumming, kneading, friction and pressure strokes. All are very relaxing.

Meditation is a self-help technique in which the power of concentration is used to control thoughts and to calm the body. Those experienced in meditation enter a trance-like state and some can lower their pulse and blood pressure at will. Muscular tension drops, circulation improves and brain wave patterns change. Meditation often leads to sleep.

Naturopathy is based on the belief that the body can heal itself, given the right conditions. Naturopaths use vitamins, minerals, dietary changes (e.g. fasting), hydrotherapy, relaxation techniques and sometimes manipulation. Many are trained in osteopathy. Naturopaths aim to identify the underlying cause of illness rather than merely relieve the symptoms. Naturopathy is particularly effective against degenerative diseases such as arthritis and emphysema.

Reflexology originated in China more than 5,000 years ago. The

Ancient Egyptians also used the technique. Reflexology is based on the principle that points (reflexes) in the feet are indirectly related to distant parts of the body. Massage and tiny pressure movements over these reflexes stimulate distant areas and organs to relieve symptoms. The presence of tenderness and subtle textural changes in the feet are diagnostic of certain illnesses.

Shiatsu is a form of Japanese massage. Practitioners use their fingers, thumbs, palms, forearms, elbows, and sometimes knees or feet to stimulate pressure points. These lie over energy lines through which the life force (Qi) is thought to flow. The abdomen (Hara) is thought to be the centre of the life force and the abdomen may be stimulated as well as another part of the body (e.g. inner thigh) to stimulate energy flow.

Thalassotherapy is a form of hydrotherapy based on the healing properties of sea water and seaweed. Seaweed extracts are added to baths or used as body wraps and poultices to encourage sweating and to draw impurities out of the skin. Seaweed is rich in trace elements and minerals, some of which are absorbed by the skin. People who are allergic to iodine should avoid this therapy.

Tissue salts are present through the body. Some homoeopaths believe that 12 tissue salts are vital for health and that depletion of these causes illness. Tissue salts are given to correct a mineral deficiency or relative imbalances. Different salts are helpful for different menstrual problems:

- kali phos – for premenstraul syptoms, heavy periods or depression
- silica – for heavy periods
- nat mur – for fluid retention
- nat suplh – for fluid retention
- mag phos – for painful periods.

Tablets are lactose-based and are not suitable for those with a milk-sugar intolerance.

Visualisation techniques rely on the power of suggestion and positive thought to harness mind-over-matter phenomena. By visualising a desired, positive outcome (e.g. good health, self-confidence, tumour regression) the person can achieve self-awareness and self-healing. Those using the technique literally picture their way to health.

Yoga is an oriental technique that involves postural exercises, breathing techniques and relaxation. It is excellent for improving joint suppleness and relieving stress.

Relaxation

Relaxation helps to switch off your body's stress responses and to overcome pain. The following is a simple relaxation exercise that you may find helpful:

Find somewhere quiet and warm to lie down. Remove your shoes and loosen tight clothing. You are going to work round your body, tensing and relaxing different muscle groups to relieve tension. Close your eyes and keep them closed throughout the relaxation exercise.

First, lift your **forearms** into the air, bend them at the elbow and clench your fists hard. Concentrate only on the tension in these muscles.

Breathe in deeply and slowly. As you breathe out, start to relax and let the tension in your arms drain away. Release your clenched fists and lower your arms gently down beside you. Feel the tension flow out of them until your fingers start to tingle. Your arms may start to feel as though they don't belong to you. Keep breathing gently and slowly.

Now tense your **shoulders and neck**, shrugging your shoulders up as high as you can. Feel the tension in your head, shoulders, neck and chest. Hold it for a moment. Then, slowly let the tension flow away. Breathe gently and slowly as the tension flows away.

Now lift your **head** up and push it forwards. Feel the tension in your neck. Tighten all your **facial muscles**. Clench your teeth, frown and screw up your eyes. Feel the tension on your face, the tightness in your skin and jaw, the wrinkles on your brow. Hold this tension for a few seconds then start to relax. Let go gradually, concentrating on each set of muscles as they relax. A feeling of warmth will spread across your head as the tension is released. Your head will feel heavy and very relaxed.

Continue in this way, working next on your **back** muscles (provided you don't have a back problem) by pulling your shoulders and head backwards and arching your back upwards. Hold this for a few moments before letting your weight sink comfortably down as you relax. Check that your arms, head and neck are still relaxed too.

Pull in your **abdomen** as tightly as you can. Then, as you breathe out, slowly release and feel the tension drain away. Now blow out your stomach as if tensing against a blow. Hold this tension for a few moments, then slowly relax. Make sure tension has not crept back into parts of your body you have already relaxed. Your upper body should feel heavy, calm and relaxed.

Now, concentrate on your **legs**. Pull your **toes** up towards you and feel the tightness down the front of your legs. Push your toes away from you and feel the tightness spread up your legs. Hold this for a few moments, then lift your legs into the air, either together or one at a time. Hold for a few moments and then lower your legs until they are at rest.

Relax your thighs, buttocks, calves and feet. Let them flop under their own weight and relax. Feel the tension flow down your legs and out through your toes. Feel your legs become heavy and relaxed. Your toes may tingle.

Your whole body should now feel very heavy and very relaxed. Breathe calmly and slowly and feel all that tension drain away. Imagine you are lying on a warm, sunny beach with gentle ocean waves rolling in beside you. Relax for at least twenty minutes, occasionally checking your body for tension.

In your own time bring the session to a close. Count slowly backwards from 5 to 1, then clench your fists as tight as you can and relax. Repeat this and then rub your hands together until they feel warm.

Cover your eyes with your warm hands and open them into the dark space. Remove your hands and accustom yourself to the light. Roll over onto your side and, when ready, sit up and enjoy the feeling.

Progressive relaxation is widely used as a method of reducing tension. The technique is easy to understand and suits most people. It does need regular practice, but some positive results are felt almost immediately.

· *Describing your pain* ·

You need to describe your pain as exactly as possible to your doctor, so that he or she can assess what is causing it. Have a look at the check list below and choose the most apt descriptions for the pain(s) you experience. Note that there may be more than one type of pain at different times of the month.

Pain descriptions

aching
gnawing
dragging
throbbing
stabbing
burning
stinging
bruising
sharp
dull
crushing
tight
constant

comes and goes in waves
colicky
deep
superficial

worse or better on breathing in
worse or better on leaning forwards
worse, better or triggered by eating
worse, better or triggered on opening bowels
worse, better or triggered on starting menstruation
radiates (spreads) to elsewhere on the body

Which painkillers make it better?
Which painkillers don't touch it?

Then decide how bad your pain is, on a scale of 1–10.
where: 1 is a little twinge
        10 is the worst pain you could ever imagine.

Try marking on the line below how severe your pain is

1	5	10

· *Charting your symptoms* ·

An important part of any self-help programme is charting your symptoms. This lets you give your doctor accurate information about your symptoms, rather than vaguely remembered impressions.

Make up a chart similar to the one on page 178 (or photocopy this one) and fill it out for at least two months, preferably three or more. This will let your doctor see exactly how bad your symptoms are.

In the column for each day:

- Shade in the days in which you have your period.
- Fill in which symptoms you experience using the following code:

    0 = none   √ = mild   * = moderate   ! = severe

Telling endometriosis and fibroids apart

Feature	Endometriosis	Fibroids
severe pain	yes	no
deep pain during sex	yes	possibly
subfertility	yes	possibly
pelvic mass	possibly	yes
pelvic nodules	yes	no
ultrasound confirms	no	yes

MONTH

DAY OF MONTH

Symptom	1 2 3 4 5 6 7 8 9 10 11 12 13 14 15 16 17 18 19 20 21 22 23 24 25 26 27 28 29 30 31
premenstrual pain	
painful periods	
mild pain	
moderate pain	
severe pain	
pain mid-cycle	
pain at any time	
painful sex	
low back pain	
pain in inner thighs	
ache or pain elsewhere	
spotting	
loss of stale brown blood	
heavy bleeding	
loss of large cloths	
swollen abdomen	
bloated feeling	
abdominal tenderness	
painful bowel motions	
diarrhoea	
constipation	
rectal bleeding	
nausea	
vomiting	
urinary frequency	
pain on passing water	
blood in urine	
dizziness	
feeling hot and cold	
headache	
pain stopping sleep	
insomnia	
irritability	
depression	
unusual bruising	
coughing up blood	
other	

GLOSSARY

Adenomyosis The presence of endometrial tissue within the wall of the uterus.

Analogue A substance that resembles something else

Anovulatory cycles Menstrual cycles in which an egg is not released.

Anteverted Tilted forwards eg an anteverted womb.

Carcinoma A type of cancer.

Corpus luteum The yellow coloured cysts that forms once an ovarian follicle has released its egg and collapsed in on itself.

Cortex The tissues that form the outer part of an organ eg ovarian cortex.

Dysmenorrhoea Painful periods.

Dysuria Painful urination.

Ectopic Occurring outside its normal site eg an ectopic pregnancy is one occuring outside the womb.

Endometrioma An endometrial cyst on the ovary.

Follicle An egg-containing nest of cells, of which there are hundreds of thousands in each ovary.

FSH Follicle stimulating hormone, which is released from the pituitary gland to act on the ovary.

Fundus The upper part of the body of the uterus, which lies between the Fallopian tubes.

Gonadotrophins Hormones that act on the gonads (ovaries or testicles) eg LH, FSH, hCG.

hCG Human chorionic gonadotrophin, a hormone released by the developing placenta in early pregnancy. hCG is detected in pregnancy tests.

Infarct Death of a tissue due to poor blood supply and lack of oxygen.

Intramural Within a wall eg intramural fibroid within the wall of the uterus.

Lesion An area of disease – eg a patch of ectopic endometrial tissue.

LH Leutinising hormone, which is released from the pituitary gland to act on the ovary.

Lumen The hollow of an organ or tube.

Macrophage A scavenger cell that absorbs and destroys cell debris and invading organisms.

Medulla The tissues that form the inner part of an organ eg ovarian medulla.

Metaplasia The changing of a cell or tissue into another type of cell or tissue.

Myoma Another word for a fibroid.

Oogenesis The egg-forming process within a female embryo.

Peritoneum (peritoneal membrane) The membrane lining the abdominal cavity and forming a covering for the abdominal and pelvic organs.

Pituitary gland A gland at the base of the brain which secretes several hormones, two of which (FSH, LH) are important in the menstrual cycle.

Prolactin A hormone released from the pituitary gland that acts on the breast to stimulate milk production.

Retroverted Tilted backwards eg a retroverted uterus.

Stroma A tissue that forms the framework and covering of an organ.

Useful Addresses — UK

Please send a stamped, self-addressed envelope if writing to any organisation for information leaflets.

Endometriosis

National Endometriosis Society
Suite 50, Westminster Palace Gardens
1–7 Artillery Row
London SW1T 1RR

Tel: 0171-222 2781
Helpline: 0171-222 2781

Support for sufferers. Newsletter, leaflet, reading list, booklets. Crisis support line 7pm–10pm

Diet

Centre for Pregnancy Nutrition
The University of Sheffield
Dept. of Obstetrics and Gynaecology
Clinical Sciences Centre
Northern General Hospital
Herries Road
Sheffield S5 7AU

Well woman and gynaecology clinics

Marie Stopes
108 Whitfield Street
London W1P 6BE

Tel: 0171 388 4843

Family Planning

Family Planning Information Service
27–35 Mortimer Street
London W1N 7RJ

Tel: 0171 837 5432

Natural Family Planning Centre
Birmingham Maternity Hospital
Queen Elizabeth Medical Centre
Edgbaston
Birmingham B15 2TG

Send an SAE and a request for leaflets or the name of a teacher in your area.

Pregnancy

Foresight
28 The Paddock
Godalming
Surrey GU7 1XD

Advice on preconceptual care, recurrent miscarriage, infertility. Private general health checks. Dietary advice. Leaflets; books.

Miscarriage Association
Clayton Hospital
Northgate
Wakefield WF1 3JF

Tel: 01924 200799

Support and advice to women and families experiencing miscarriage. Leaflets; newsletter.

Infertility

Child
Charter House
43 St. Leonard's Road
Bexhill-on-Sea
TN40 1JA

Tel: 01424 732361

Advice and support for those having difficulty conceiving. Promotes research into infertility.

ISSUE – National Fertility Association
114 Lichfield Street
Walsall WS1 1SZ

Tel: 01922 793225

Information and support for infertile couples who are members of the association.

British Pregnancy Advisory Service
Austy Manor
Wootton Wauen
Solihull,
West Midlands B95 6BX

Counselling and referral for termination of pregnancy.

The London Women's Clinic
113–115 Harley Street
London W1N 1DG

Tel: 0171 487 5050

Assisted conception and gynaecological Services (DI insemination)

Women's Health Concern
93–99 Upper Richmond Road
London SW15 2TG

Tel: 0181 780 3916
Helpline: 0181 780 3007

Advice and counselling on all kinds of gynaecological problems including infertility, menopause and HRT.

INDEX